Fine Dining
PRISON COOKBOOK 3

100 Ways to Satisfy Your Taste
And Inspire Your Day

Troy Traylor

Freebird Publishers

North Dighton, MA

Freebird Publishers
221 Pearl St., 541, North Dighton, MA 02764
Info@FreebirdPublishers.com
www.FreebirdPublishers.com

Copyright © 2023
Fine Dining Prison Cookbook 3
By Troy Traylor

All rights reserved. No part of this book may be reproduced in any form or by any means without the Publisher's prior written consent, except in brief quotes used in reviews.

All Freebird Publishers titles, imprints, and distributed lines are available at special quantity discounts for bulk purchases for sales promotions, premiums, fundraising, educational, or institutional use.

ISBN: 978-1-952159-44-2

Printed in the United States of America

Dedicated to:

Troy Neal Traylor, Jr.

Madeline Emma Traylor

and all my loyal readers.

Acknowledgments

Jesus Christ: I sincerely thank and praise you for leading me to find meaning and purpose in this life. It is only due to your love and mercy that I have the means and ability to write books and encourage others. I find hope and strength in you and you alone.

Bonnie & Danny Cantrell: I thank you and love you both so much. Your belief in me and your continual support is a true blessing. You have loved me until I could love myself, and I owe you so much gratitude. May joy and happiness continue to fill you both.

Kelsey Eiland: You have become the little sister I never had. I have never met another human being as compassionate and dedicated as you are. I could never repay you for the years of love and encouragement you have shared with me. You have left me speechless by the amount of help and patience you exhibit. I want to thank you for being you.

Natalie DeMarcus: It would be impossible to describe how beautiful your soul is. Over the past few years, you have helped me see who I am and what I am capable of. Good, bad, and rough times have been learning times for me. You are such a gift to my life, and I wholeheartedly cherish what we share. I love you and respect you in all ways. Thank you for sharing this life and journey with me. I may be "flippin' crazy," but when you know, you know.

I would also like to acknowledge and thank the countless others who have taken the time to share tips, recipes, and peace of mind with me. There are too many of you to list by name; I want to say thanks because I doubt my books would even exist without each of you. I wish everyone a life of peace and happiness. My prayers are with each of you.

Preface

This is the third and final book in the Fine Dining series. In my last book on cooking, I want to share some more delicious recipes and vital knowledge on products and nutrition.

Eating healthy today is essential, let alone in prison. Prison food is full of starch and many other things that will harm the body over a long period of time.

With all the healthier choices of eating we now see on TV, some of us do not have that option or the means. So, exercise is most important. You should develop an exercise routine in prison or the free world. Some are better than none.

Wellness starts from within, and what is a better time to throw out the old unhealthy lifestyle and bring in new wholesome energy than now? Let's look at it like Spring cleaning. Spring cleaning is not finally deciding to wipe up the dust bunnies under your bunk or in the corner of your living area or living room. Spring cleaning is a time to focus on a thorough clean-up. For foodies, Spring cleaning is a time to focus on your mind, body, and soul.

Unit commissaries and local markets are now beginning to offer healthier choices. They are beginning to embrace the opportunities to provide various options that will help nourish your journey to a better and healthier holistic lifestyle.

I urge you to begin to focus on the food. You have a choice, and let us start to make healthier choices on what we put into our bodies—healthier food and snacks, healthier beverages, low-sodium options, and sugar-free options. Change does and will make a difference in how you feel and think.

I want to tell you to be mindful of your health by reviewing the Nutrition Facts and the serving size you are making. Don't just dig into your favorite snack or go-to recipes before investigating what you are eating.

Love yourself and love your health. You do not have to deprive yourself necessarily. Just be more cautious about the amounts you take in and your exercise routine. The goal of healthier living is to burn more calories than you take in.

In this third and final book, you can learn a lot. This book is about mind, body, and soul. I pray you enjoy all the recipes you try and the additional information you will read. There are page-by-page encouraging quotes as well as facts on foods. You will also find some exercise tips as well.

I thank everyone for their interest in my book(s) and encourage everyone to share this book with a dear friend or loved one.

Table of Contents

Acknowledgments iv

Preface v

Table of Contents 1

Discipline 7

Supplies Needed – Inside/Outside 9

Total Body Workout 10

What to Know About Immunity 12

Section 1: A Few Tasty Drinks 14

Convict Cold Coffee 15

Iced Donkey Punch 16

Minty Hot Cocoa 17

Tasty Hot Tea 18

White Chocolate Peppermint Cappuccino 19

Food Facts 20

Section 2: Condiments 24

Fire Mustard 25

Homemade Honey Mustard 26

Wait! So Butter is Okay Now? 27

What the latest science says about saturated fats. 27

Section 3: Dips and Sauces 29

Amazing Apple Dip 30

Bean Dip... 31

Hazelnut Crunch 32

More-Gooder Sauce 33

Ten Ways to Get More Fiber 34

Section 4: Biscuits and Muffins 37

Amazing Veggie Biscuits 38

Cheesy Corn Muffins 39

Chicken Biscuits... 40

Chicken Biscuits 2... 41

Jalapeno Biscuits 42

Jalapeno-Cheesy Corn Muffins 43

Raisin Spice Biscuits.. 44

Food Facts.. 45

Section 5: Sides 47

Bold Stuffed Peppers... 48

Pickle Boat... 49

Ranch Style Bacon 50

Red Rice 51

Sweet Fiery Rice 52

Genius Granola Hacks... 53

Bags to Buy.. 54

Two Helpful Tips... 55

Food Facts 57

Food Facts 61

Section 6: Meals of All Kinds 63
Baltimore's Bagin' Burrito 64
Cheesy Vegan Pasta 65
Chicken-Chili Taquitos 66
Chickles 67
Chili Cheese Soup 68
Chili Cheese Soupy Soup 69
Chinese Anyone 70
Chinese Chicken 71
Cowboy Tacos 72
Creamy Chicken for Two 73
EZ Cheezy Tuna Delight 74
Fabulous Fish Balls 75
Four Cheese Potato Meat Delight 76
Freaked Out Fluffy Potatoes 77
Garbage Can Rice 78
Get-Er-Done-Ramen 79
Gluten-Free Shindig 80
Hungry Mans Belt-Busting Tacos 81
Meaty Shells and Cheese 82
Pork Skin-Tuna Delight 83
Powerball Oatmeal Express 84
Prison Pazole 85
Salmon Cold Wraps 86
Someone Say Queso 87

Spicy Rice 88

Stuffed Fish Balls 89

Stuffed Pork 90

Sweet Treat Chicken 91

Traditional Tamales 92

Tuna Lasagna 94

Tuna-Mack-Cocktail 95

Typical Bean Burritos 96

Wacky-Delish-Sandwich 97

(Vegan) Cheese, Please! 98

History of Pizza 100

Food Facts 102

Section 7: Sweets and Treats 106

Baltimore's Bon Bons 107

Chocolate Brownies 108

Chocolate Éclair Soup 109

Cookie Bars Delight 110

Cookie and Cream Bars 111

Cranberry Crumble Pie 112

Excellent Empanadas 113

Felon Fruitcake 114

Holiday Cheesecake 115

Kiwi-Strawberry-Delight 116

No Bake Chocolate Raisin Nut Cookies 117

Oh-So-Good-Pie 118

O M G Reese's Replica 119

One-of-a-Kind Cheesecake 120

Peanut Butter Cream Delight 121

Pineapple Cream Pie 122

Rocky Road Parfait 123

Spicy Nut Mix 124

Strawberry-Chocolate Pie 125

Section 8: 25 Healthy Choices for the Outside: from the Inside 126

Baked Feta Spinach-Artichoke Dip 127

Black Bean and Butternut Squash Enchiladas 128

Cashew Chicken Lettuce Wraps 130

Cheesesteak Salad 132

Cheesy Cauliflower and Sweet Potato Chowder 133

Chicken Puttanesca 135

Chicken Stew with Collard Greens and Peanuts 136

Chili and Garlic Hasselback Squash 138

Cornmeal Crusted Shrimp with Corn and Okra 139

Fish Tacos Preserved Grapefruit Salsa 141

Ginger Chicken & Vegetable Noodle Soup 142

Grilled Strawberry Salsa Fresca 144

Mini Vegan Chocolate Tarts 145

Preserved Citrus Paste 146

Preserved Lemon and Fennel Roast Chicken 147

Red Lentil Soup with Saffron 149

Roasted Strawberry Frozen Yogurt 150

Roast Salmon with Kumquat -Pineapple Chutney 151

Saffranskaka (Saffron Cake) 153

Saffron Chicken Forma 155

Seven-Layer Chicken Burrito.. 157

Small-Batch Crispy Chocolate Chip Cookies................................... 158

Smoked Trout Potato Salad 159

Southwest Chopped Salad with Tomatillo Dressing........................ 160

Tofu Cauliflower & Sweet Potato Green Curry 162

Focus on the Food 163

Weather Watch... 166

Closing 169

Your Shopping List... 170

Conversion Chart.. 174

Discipline

Discipline is just consistently doing what we know we are supposed to do. I know that seems simple to say, and there is a paradox in writing that from any incarcerated resident. County jail, state, or federal prison, this applies to you. If you are not in one of these prisons or types of incarceration but in a self-made prison, this also applies to you.

Most of us are not incarcerated for doing what we are supposed to do. Some may be innocent but find themselves on the wrong end of the stick. With, like most traits, discipline can be built and strengthened.

Where many get frustrated is attempting to adhere to the strictest of regimens and setting unrealistic goals.

"I'm going to eat only peanuts and straight fish products-nothing else." Two days later, you're sick of dieting.

Or "I'm going to do two hours a day of straight burpees, seven days a week for six months." Five days go by, your joints hurt, and you look at your next workout as a punishment.

Or "I need to catch up on time lost in prison, make a million dollars, so I got to hustle in the streets." A year goes by after release, and you're fighting another case in the county jail.

Discipline means consistency in good habits, not extreme ones. Sound practices are simple, with good results.

- Be active most days.
- Eat more healthy food than you do junk.
- Do not poison yourself with drugs.
- Stay away from people and situations that have problems or unnecessary drama.
- Be productive and positive every chance you can.

It makes it easier to be disciplined if we understand how our actions are related to the end goal through inaction-that there are "more important" things than doing what needs to be done.

In those times, I often remind myself, "If it's not me, then who is going to do what needs to be done for me and those I care about?" The answer: Nobody! Taking care of "life" is what we do.

We all have something inside of us that can push us. We all have an inner animal. A warrior. Some desire to live and live better than we are at this moment. You want to be able to lift small grandchildren when you get out at 100 years old. Have you taken the time to figure out how to stay out of the infirmary and pill window? For those outside, that would be how to stay off medications and avoid doctor visits for health issues. We all must educate ourselves about preventing diabetes, high blood pressure, and high cholesterol, among many other health issues that could be avoided with self-discipline and regular exercise. If you want a change in your life and a chance to have a home outside of prison, you must prove to yourself that you are the only person who can do that. You can and will succeed if you are disciplined and show up and do what you should.

You don't have to be the greatest; you only must be good. Every small goal you set and stick to builds discipline and the foundation for bigger goals.

Supplies Needed – Inside/Outside

Inside	Outside
Large & Small Spread Bowls	Large & Small Mixing Bowls
12-ounce Coffee Mug	Same
Insert Cup	16 oz thick plastic cup
Hot Pot	Coffee Kettle
Empty Peanut Butter Jar	Same
Large and Small Chip Bags	Same
Rice Bags	Same
Old Newspaper	Same
Cream Cookie Trays	Oreo Cookie Trays (3-row)
Plastic Trash Bags	Same
ID Card	Knife
Desire	Same
Patience	Same
Passion	Same
Appetite	Same
Commissary Spoon	Tablespoon and Teaspoon

You'll need all your normal cooking items for all those outside interested in cooking from Section VIII recipes.

Total Body Workout

I will find a balance between appreciating what I have and working on what I want.

It is advisable that before any workout, you spend 5 to 10 minutes stretching. Here are a few suggestions, but there are many others you can make. Just figure out what works best for you.

Many people experience lower back pain in their lives. Some of this is due to not correctly working your erector spinae. So, to begin, lie flat on the floor on your stomach, stretch your hands out over your head, fingers fully extended, legs stretched out, toes pointed down. Now, you want to lift your hands off the ground about 6 inches and do the same with your legs/feet. Your body will resemble a banana. Hold this for three good, long breaths, in/out. Relax and repeat this exercise 10 times.

The rest of your stretching can be 5 sets of toe touches, right hand to left, and left hand to right. Hands-on hips and twist right/left 10 times each is one set. Do five sets of this. Hands above your head and lean backward, hold three deep breaths. Allow for ten sets of this.

You can feel free to add your twist to the workout routine, so these are just some ideas to help you get started.

1) **Walking Lunge:** Stand straight up and place your hands on your hips. Move your right foot forward as you would take a step. As you do this, you lean somewhat forward, and your left knee will touch the ground. Repeat the next step with your left foot, allowing the right knee to touch the ground. Do this five times for each leg (step). Ten will be 1 set. You should do 3 sets of 10.
2) **Push-ups:** We all know what a push-up is, but to work out the chest completely, you should do one set of 10 regular, one set of 10 inclines, and one set of 10

declines. That is a full set. 10 sets are recommended. Total of 300 push-ups.

3) **Squats:** Stand straight up with feet apart about as wide as your shoulders. Keep your back straight, head staring straight ahead, and bend at the knees like you're about to sit on a bucket. Now, back up to a standing position. That is one complete squat. Starting, you should be able to do three sets of 10.

4) **Sit-ups:** A blanket or mat is best to lie on. Lay flat on your back, knees bent, with approximately one foot's space between your feet and your tailbone. It is best to put your toes under something stationary, so your feet don't move. Hands behind your head. Now rise and touch your right elbow to your left knee, then lower yourself back down to the floor and repeat, touching your left elbow to the right knee. That is one complete set. You should do 50 sets. That is 100 sit-ups.

You're almost done. Now pick two exercises and complete one full exercise, immediately followed by the other. This is called a superset and adds a cardiovascular element to the workout.

This is enough to get you started, but not overwhelming. Feel free to increase repetitions to accommodate fitness levels.

And one last thing: since this is new to you and you want to be sure this will not cause you any injuries, please consult your physician before you attempt these exercises.

Cardio is also good for the body. Running in place, jumping jacks, and walking up stairs are good sources. The goal is to burn more calories than you ingest. A tip to know when you're burning calories: if you are exercising and sweating, you're burning calories. Good luck, and stay focused.

What to Know About Immunity

Keeping your body's inner army strong can help guard against the common cold, flu, and COVID-19. Here's what will and won't boost your immune system.

TRUE

Your body's defenses weaken with age. Research shows that as more candles top your birthday cake, the immune function begins to decline, leaving adults over 65 years of age more vulnerable to severe illness from viral and bacterial infections. (There's a scientific term for this process: immunosenescence.) You have fewer circulating immune cells, and changes to those you do have make them slower to respond to infectious invaders. To bolster your defenses, exercise regularly, eat a well-balanced diet, avoid smoking and drinking too much alcohol, and stay current on vaccines.

MOSTLY TRUE

Probiotics boost immune function. The microbiome plays a vital role in a strong, resilient immune system. A recent review found that probiotic supplements (which contain strains of "good" gut bacteria) decreased the risk of becoming sick with a respiratory infection and shortened its duration among those who did come down with one. Probiotics may activate immune cells that fight viruses, reduce inflammation, and kick out "bad" bacteria in your GI system that could open the door to illness. However, this mechanism isn't fully understood, and higher-quality clinical studies are needed. Plus, the benefits may only apply to specific strains of bacteria, and probiotics are not necessarily effective.

MOSTLY FALSE

A megadose of C can squash a cold. This vitamin does play an important role in immune function. But at the first sign of sniffles, don't run to the drugstore to load up on C-high dose supplements. They won't prevent or shorten the duration of a cold, according to a review published in Frontiers in Immunity. (Plus, your body can absorb only so much vitamin C in one sitting; you'll simply urinate out any excess.) Some exceptions: Competitive athletes (intense physical stress can lower immunity) and those with metabolic disorders or heart disease may want to take up to 1 gram of vitamin C daily; groups are more susceptible to viral infections and may benefit from an extra boost of C, the review notes. Everyone else can skip the supplement and opt for C-rich foods instead, like strawberries, bell peppers, kiwi, broccoli, citrus, and potatoes.

FALSE

Sleep has little impact on immunity. Rest is one of the top recommendations for recovering from a cold, but it's also vital to prevent it. Immune function is closely tied to sleep, circadian rhythms (your body's internal clock), and inadequate shuteye can make you more susceptible to infection. In one experimental study, participants who got less than 6 hours of sleep a night for one week were four times more likely to get sick after exposure to a cold virus than those who got at least 7 hours. Other research has found that adequate rest may improve immune response following vaccinations—just one more reason to get more ZZs.

"My greatest strength in life is my drive. Explore what you're naturally good at, and get the tools and teachings to be even better."

Section 1:
A Few Tasty Drinks

Convict Cold Coffee

Ingredients
2 heaping Tbsp. cappuccino of choice
3 pkgs. Sweetener (sub 6 tsp. sugar)
½ coffee mug hot water
½ coffee mug cold water
1 level Tbsp. Columbian coffee
1 coffee mug of ice

Directions
Set the ice aside until the end. In a coffee mug, combine cappuccino, coffee, sweeteners, and hot water. Stir until all is dissolved. Now add cold water, stir again, and pour over ice. That's how we convicts do it!

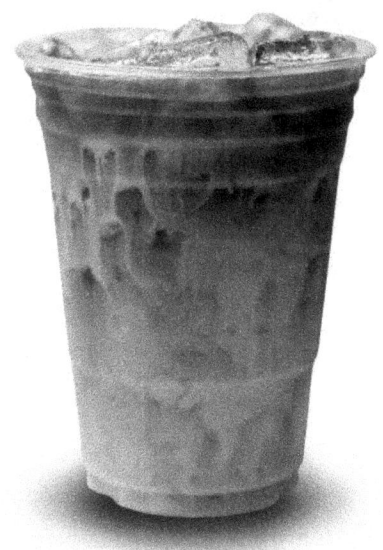

Today, tell yourself;
I give thanks to
and dance with the
flow of my life.

Iced Donkey Punch

Ingredients
1 (12 oz.) can strawberry-kiwi juice
1 pkg blue typhoon drink mix
2 Tbsp. hot sauce
2 good mugs of ice
1 (12 oz.) can Sprite
2 fireball candies (crushed)
1 large spread bowl

Directions
Set the ice aside until the end. Combine all ingredients in a large spread bowl and stir until all drink mix is dissolved. Add ice and drink it up! Nice fruity drink with a kick.

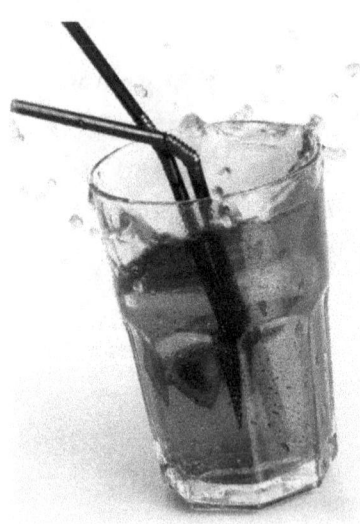

Today, tell yourself:
My trust in myself and in life is
constantly increasing, everything
It is as it should be.

Minty Hot Cocoa

Ingredients
4 heaping Tbsp. hot chocolate mix
1 level spoonful of coffee
1 coffee mug of hot water
1 (1 oz.) mint stick (crushed)
2 Tbsp. creamer

Directions
Combine all ingredients in your coffee mug and stir until the mint stick is fully dissolved. This is as easy as it gets. Drink up!

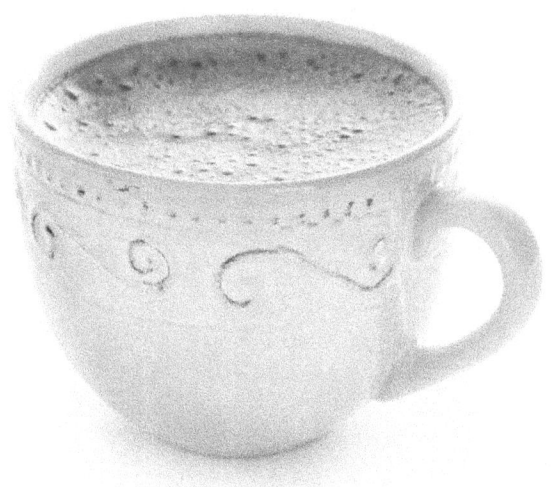

Today, tell yourself:
I will only focus on what I
can control and let go of the rest.

Tasty Hot Tea

Ingredients
4 (1 oz.) mint sticks
8 sweeteners (sub 10 tsp. sugar)
8 tea bags
4 individual fireballs
1 (12 oz.) cranberry juice
4 coffee mugs hot water

Directions
Crush up all candies. Equally, divide all ingredients into 4 coffee mugs. Stir until all candies are melted. That's it, invite a few associates and drink up—a great way to begin the day.

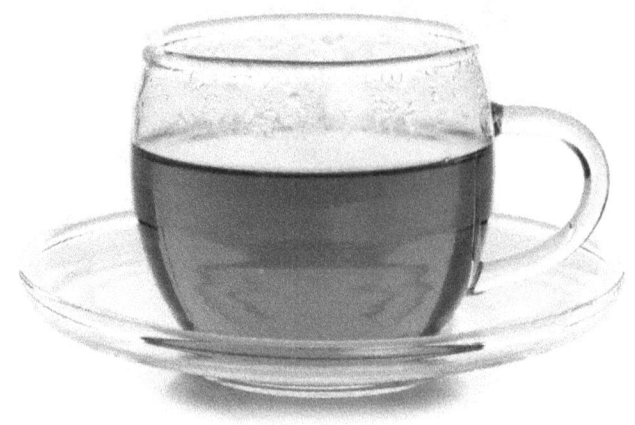

Today, tell yourself:
This is the day to begin my journey
to evolve into a better person, friend
and members of my community.

White Chocolate Peppermint Cappuccino

Ingredients
1 coffee mug hot water
3 Tbsp. hot chocolate mix
1 (1 oz.) mint stick
1 tsp. cheap coffee
4 Tbsp. vanilla cappuccino
2 Tbsp. instant milk
1 tsp. Columbian coffee
1 tsp. sweetener (sub 2 tsp. sugar)

Directions
Heat water in a hot pot. The hotter the pot, the better. Pour a half mug of water into your mug. Now stir in cappuccino, hot chocolate mix, and instant milk. Crush the mint stick and add it to the mug, along with the remaining ingredients, and stir until the mint stick is fully dissolved. Fill the mug the rest of the way with hot water, stir again, and drink up.

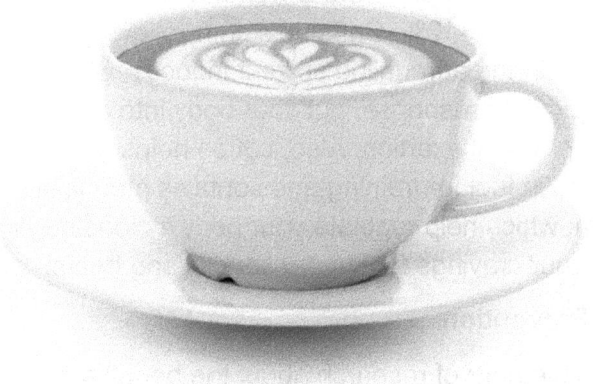

Today, tell yourself:
I have been blessed with unique abilities
and I see value in myself.

Food Facts

Coffee and Tea

What's Up with Caffeine?

Both coffee and tea contain large amounts of caffeine, a mild stimulant that provides heightened mental capacity and creativity, boosts physical energy, and relieves pain. However, people who are sensitive to caffeine can experience several negative side effects, such as insomnia, anxiety, or irritability. Excessive caffeine consumption can cause irregular heartbeat, eye pressure that can lead to glaucoma, and even calcium loss through the urine, which can lead to osteoporosis. Yet a moderate intake of either coffee or tea as part of your day-to-day regimen has been consistently associated with a reduced risk of several chronic diseases. As with anything, moderation is key.

For Exercise

A cup of coffee an hour before a workout improves your performance by 11-12%. Caffeine's pain-relieving properties, combined with the adrenaline spike it induces, which induces your fight or flight response, put your body into a state where it thrives on physical exertion. Also, coffee helps break down fat cells for use in fuel for training and contains magnesium and potassium, which help regulate your body's blood sugar levels and curb your cravings for sugary snacks and treats.

Disease Prevention

There is a plethora of research about the benefits of coffee and tea for your long-term health. Such facts have been unearthed that a coffee drinker's risk of premature death is 25% lower than that of those who don't imbibe daily.
Consumption of 2-3 cups of coffee daily is associated with a lower stroke risk and a 20% reduced risk of prostate cancer. It also may prevent the most common type of skin cancer: basal

cell carcinoma. Coffee consumption reduces your risk of dementia; high levels of caffeine in the bloodstream curbs the threat of Alzheimer's. Caffeine elevates a few neurotransmitters that boost your mood, and studies have shown that just two cups of coffee a day prevent the risk of suicide by 50%.

Coffee or Tea?

For most, it is a matter of taste. Both provide a wide swath of health benefits and are consumed in large amounts regularly in various parts of the world.

Consensus

Be aware that caffeine consumption is a habit that can be either good or bad. Excessive amounts of sugar to combat the sometimes-bitter qualities of both beverages can work against their benefits. Most doctors suggest that if you don't already have a coffee or tea habit, don't pick one up.

Source: Wikipedia.org

Refined Sugar

How Much is Okay?

It's hard to say since sugar is not required as a nutrient in your diet. The Institute of Medicine, which sets Recommended Dietary Allowances, or RDAs, has not issued a formal number for sugar. However, the American Heart Association suggests that men consume no more than 150 calories per day (about 6 teaspoons) of added sugar daily. That is close to the amount in a 12-ounce can of soda.

Did You Know?

Americans average about 270 calories of sugar daily, about 17 teaspoons a day.

Added Sugar

Added sugar is sugar that food manufacturers add to products to increase flavor and extend shelf life.

Food Labels

Reading food labels is one of the best ways to monitor your added sugar intake. Look for the following names for added sugar and try to avoid either or cut back on the amount or frequency of the foods where they are found: brown sugar, corn sweetener, corn syrup, fruit juice concentrate, high-fructose corn syrup, honey, inverted sugar, malt sugar, molasses, syrup sugar molecules ending in "ose" (dextrose, fructose, glucose, lactose, maltose, sucrose).

Cardiovascular Disease

The effects of added sugar intake- higher blood pressure, inflammation, weight gain, diabetes, and fatty liver disease- are all linked to an increased risk for heart attack and stroke.

Inflammation

Consuming too much added sugar can raise blood pressure and increase chronic inflammation, both pathological pathways to heart disease. Inflammation can also be the cause of joint pain and aging skin.

Your Teeth

Bacteria that cause cavities love to eat sugar that lingers in your mouth after you eat something sweet.

Impact on Health

Over the course of the 15-year study, published in 2014 in JAMA Internal Medicine, people who got 17% to 21% of their calories from added sugar had a 38% higher risk of dying from cardiovascular disease compared with those who consumed 8% of their calories as added sugar.

Eggs

When a hen lays an egg, it has a coating called the bloom. This bloom protects the egg.

Eggs with the bloom on them do not have to be refrigerated. However, if you rinse the eggs, you remove the bloom, and the eggs MUST be refrigerated. Eggs with the bloom still intact can be stored at room temperature for up to 3 months.

When you are ready to use the eggs, you'll want to float them to be sure they are still good.

To float eggs, you can use a glass cup, glass bowl, or any glass that will hold water.

Fill the container until the egg is submerged in it. If your egg lays flat at the bottom of this container, that is a good egg. If the egg stands up at the bottom of the container, that is an 'iffy' egg. And finally, if the egg floats to the top of the container, that is a bad egg.

These facts are contributed by Mrs. Shelly T.

They say, "Things get better with age."
Are you a better person today than yesterday?

Section 2:
Condiments

Fire Mustard

Ingredients
1/3 (16 oz.) bottle squeeze cheese
½ (6 oz.) bottle hot sauce
1 tsp. no-salt seasoning
1 tsp. garlic powder
1 (.14 gram) pkg. lemon-lime electrolyte
1/3 (14 oz.) bottle yellow mustard
1 (1.3 oz.) jalapeno pepper
1 tsp. onion powder
1 (.14 gram) pkg orange electrolyte

Directions
Leave enough cheese in the bottle to cover up to the middle of the first groove on the bottle. This is approx. 1/3 bottle. Now, fill the second groove with mustard. Now add your hot sauce and shake well. Dice up jalapeno pepper into small pieces, add these and the remaining ingredients to the bottle, and shake well. You want it all thoroughly mixed.
Enjoy this with sandwiches, crackers, and some spreads.

Today, tell yourself:
I am just beginning the best part of my life.

Troy Traylor

Homemade Honey Mustard

Ingredients
8 Tbsp. mustard
2 Tbsp. strawberry preserves
1 cleaned-out peanut butter jar
4 (2 oz.) pkgs. cream cheese
1 heaping Tbsp. cappuccino

Directions
Combine all ingredients in a peanut butter jar and whip well. Once all is mixed thoroughly, begin eating. You should eat within 48 hours, but this will not be hard once you taste it. Extremely good!

Today, tell yourself:
I know that whatever is meant for me is making its way to me.

Wait! So, Butter is Okay Now?

What the latest science says about saturated fats.

Fat has a long-standing identity crisis. In the '90s, all of it was bad. Later, only some types were unhealthy, while others were good. (Looking at you, avocado.) More recently, it seems like most fats are back on the table, with headlines celebrating butter, coconut oil, and other formerly vilified saturated fats. Confusing, right?

Some pro-butter news stems from several recent meta-analyses of large observational studies that found no link between saturated fat intake and heart disease. Plus, a meta-analysis of randomized controlled trials (the gold standard for research) reported inconsistent results but leaned toward a lack of association.

Despite this research, the Dietary Guidelines for Americans still recommends limiting saturated fat intake to less than 10% of your daily calories (a target that only one-quarter of Americans are hitting). Why? Because balance is important. "Saturated fats aren't intrinsically bad, but modern diets tend to deliver too much, and an excess is bad." So, there's no need to eliminate saturated fat from your diet; just don't go overboard and be mindful of what you eat instead. Now, remember that discrepancies between studies are often due to differences in the comparison or the saturated fat replacement. In other words, whether saturated fat is good, bad, or immaterial depends on what you compare it to. So now you should have a better understanding of what should replace saturated fats in the diet.

Look to unsaturated fats, as they have been shown to lower your risk of dying from cardiovascular disease. While they're all heart-healthy, a study published in the journal Nutrition Metabolism and Cardiovascular Disease found that polyunsaturated fats (soybean and corn oil are good sources), and especially omega-3 polyunsaturated fats (found in fatty fish, walnuts, and flaxseeds), are particularly beneficial.

And be careful not to trade saturated-fat-heavy foods for those added sugars or other ultra-refined carbs. Some of the best evidence suggests that saturated fats from meats and dairy are almost identically as harmful as added sugars. (That's why the fat-free craze of the '90s was such bad news: food companies stripped out both saturated and unsaturated fats and then pumped up flavor with sweeteners and other refined carbs.)

The Bottom Line: A better way of looking at this than which fats are good and which are bad: What foods make your overall diet and health better? You already know the answer: vegetables, fruits, legumes, whole grains, seafood, nuts, and seeds, all of which are not significant sources of saturated fat. Stock your locker or pantry with a variety of fats and oils for cooking (yes, even butter!). They each have unique culinary uses, and they'll provide a good mix of fatty acids in your diet.

Good intentions are great.
But they also only go so far.

Section 3:
Dips and Sauces

Amazing Apple Dip

Ingredients
1 apple
4 vanilla cream cookies
6 Tbsp. water
1 (2 oz.) bag vanilla chike (protein powder)
1 (.14 oz.) pkg. orange electrolyte
1 small spread bowl

Directions
Dice your apple into smaller size cubes. Can leave the skin on if you prefer. Combine all ingredients in a small spread bowl and stir until all ingredients are incorporated. Great on snack crackers, saltine crackers, and even flour tortillas.

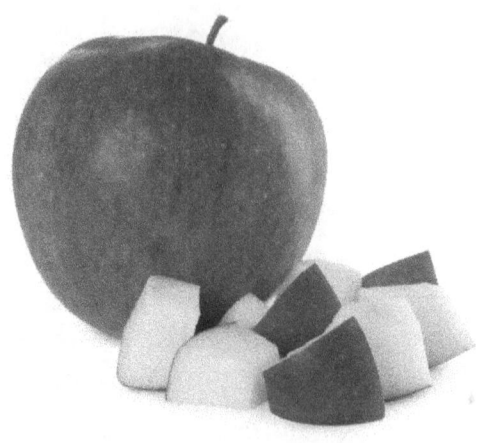

Today, tell yourself:
I am thankful for where I've been,
Happy with where I am and excited
about where I'm going.

Fine Dining Prison Cookbook 3

Bean Dip

Ingredients
½ (15 oz.) bag of refried beans
4 Tbsp. onion powder
Any other seasonings to taste
1 large spread bowl
3 coffee mugs hot water

Directions
Combine all ingredients in a large mixing bowl, stir well, cover, and allow to sit for 15 minutes. Break out your favorite chips and enjoy each bite.

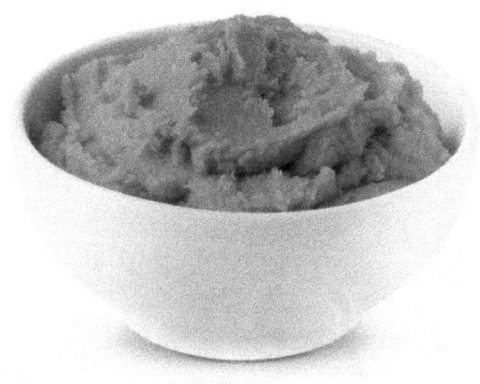

Today, tell yourself:
Every day, I am grateful to grow,
No matter how slowly.

Troy Traylor

Hazelnut Crunch

Ingredients
1 small spread bowl
5 heaping Tbsp. hazelnut spread
1 (2 oz.) pkg. energizer mix
3 Tbsp. raisin bran cereal
2 Matzo crackers (substitute saltine crackers or snack crackers)

Directions
Use a small spread bowl and combine hazelnut spread, Energizer mix, and cereal. Use a spoon to mix thoroughly. Grab your crackers and enjoy.

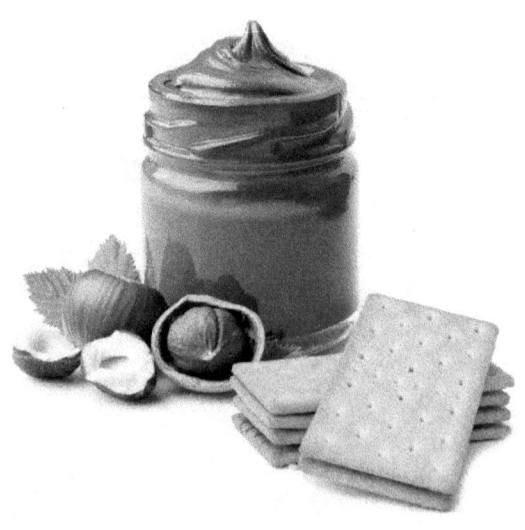

Today, tell yourself:
Each day, I discover new,
simple ways to create a life that I love.

More-Gooder Sauce

Ingredients
1 (16 oz.) bottle squeeze cheese
1 (15 oz.) jar sandwich spread
2 (6 oz.) bottles hot sauce
3 Tbsp. onion powder
1-1/2 Tbsp. garlic powder
3 Tbsp. no-salt seasoning
3 empty peanut butter jars with lids

Directions
Divide these ingredients evenly between the 3 jars, stir well, and enjoy. This sauce is good on just about everything; that's why you'll need 3 jars ;).

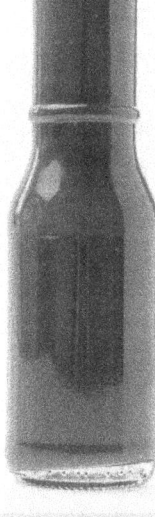

Today, tell yourself:
I will open my mind and my heart to
new opportunities and unexpected possibilities.

Ten Ways to Get More Fiber

This nutrient does so many good things for your body, from aiding weight management and quelling inflammation to protecting against heart disease and type 2 diabetes. Yet, only 7% of U.S. adults eat enough, according to a new American Society of Nutrition study. Not that we don't try. The problem is, we need lots of the stuff- 25 grams a day for women, 38 for men. To really hit your quota, you'll need a decent chunk with every meal (and snack). Check out the fiber-rich foods below, along with tricks from dietitians for adding more of them to your day.

1) Avocados (5g per 1/3 avocado)
   Avocado toast and guacamole are no-brainers, but New York-based dietitian Frances Largeman-Roth, RDN, author of Eating in Color, likes this sweet pudding option that combines avocados with fiber-rich pumpkin puree: Beat a ripe avocado with an electric mixer until creamy. Add 1 cup unseasoned pumpkin puree, ¼ cup sugar, ½ tsp. pumpkin pie spice and ½ tsp. vanilla extract. Mix until smooth, cover with plastic wrap, and refrigerate for at least 1 hour. (Makes 4 servings, 5g fiber each)
2) Beets (2g per ½ cup)
   This root veg is a nutrient powerhouse, says Breana Killeen, M.P.H., RD, Test Kitchen manager at Eating Well. In addition to fiber, beets are rich in antioxidants and contain natural nitrates, which can help lower blood pressure. Try them roasted, pickled, raw, or shaved over your next taco or salad.
3) Artichokes (5 g per ½ cup)
   Artichokes are among the highest-fiber veggies. Add canned or thawed frozen artichoke hearts to pasta, salads, or sandwiches. Or whip up a batch of baked feta spinach-artichoke dip (1g per ¼ cup).
4) Rye Crispbreads (5g per 3 crackers)
   Swap your whole-wheat crackers for these crispbreads with double the fiber. Top with hummus or guacamole,

which adds even more grams to take your snacking game to the next level.

5) Chickpeas (7g per ½ cup, cooked)
You probably know that beans are fiber superstars, but have you considered adding them to more than just soups and salads? Vancouver-based dietitian Desiree Nielsen, RD, author of Eat More Plants, suggests a breakfast chickpea "scramble": Just lightly mash cooked chickpeas in a sauté pan with olive oil and season as you would eggs.

6) Raspberries (10g per cup)
They're one of the highest-fiber fruits, and Nielsen likes to add them to a jam with chia seeds, which are also high in nutrients (3g per Tbsp.). Try simmering 2 cups of raspberries until they break down. Remove from heat and stir in 2 Tbsp. Chia seeds (they'll create a gel as the jam set). (Makes 1 cup; 3g fiber per 2 Tbsp.)

7) Popcorn (3g per 3 cups popped)
Get out the air popper or your old-timey stovetop popcorn maker and pop up some fiber-then get creative with your toppings. Try Killeen's favorite: toasted sesame oil and nutritional yeast.

8) Cocoa Powder (2g per Tbsp.)
Surprised? It's true! So, enjoy a mug of homemade hot cocoa, knowing you're getting more fiber than a slice of whole wheat bread. Whisk 2 Tbsp. unsweetened cocoa powder into a cup of warm low-fat milk, with 1 tsp. sugar. (Makes 1 serving, 4g fiber)

9) Pears (6g for 1 medium fruit)
Snack on fresh pears or poach them in cider and serve with whipped cream for a healthy dessert. You can also cook them to make your own "Pear sauce," just like the way you would applesauce, says Killeen. She recommends adding cardamom and vanilla for extra flavor.

10) Red Lentils (8g per ½ cup, cooked)

Looking for a way to eat more lentils? Try adding them to a smoothie! Aside from fiber, they also have protein that makes a drink filling enough to be a meal. "Plus, their starch provides a nice, creamy texture," says Julie Stefanski, RDN, a spokesperson for the Academy of Nutrition and Dietetics. To save time, cook a batch in bulk, cool, and store in ½ cup servings in the freezer (thaw before adding to your smoothie).

*Don't just list your values; rank them in order
of importance so they help you choose between competing
priorities-honesty versus loyalty,
freedom versus security.*

Section 4:
Biscuits and Muffins

Troy Traylor

Amazing Veggie Biscuits

Ingredients
1 serving-preferred veggies from tray
2 sleeves saltine crackers
2 rolls snack crackers
1/3 (16 oz.) bag tortilla chips
3 (1.375 oz.) pkgs. cheese and chive snack crackers
1/3 coffee mug hot water
3 spicy vegetable seasonings
1 large spread bowl
1-2 rice bags

Directions
Dice vegetables and crush all crackers and chips. Dissolve seasonings in 1/3 of a coffee mug of hot water. Now, combine all ingredients in a large spread bowl and quickly mix well. Let it sit, covered, for 30 minutes. Divide the mixture into 6-8 equal parts and form your biscuits. Let sit for another 10 minutes, then 2 at a time; place in a rice bag and set the bag down in a hot pot to heat for 1-1/2 hours. Two hot pots are best for this. This could be biscuits or burgers, if burgers are put on bread or flour tortillas and topped with your favorite condiments.

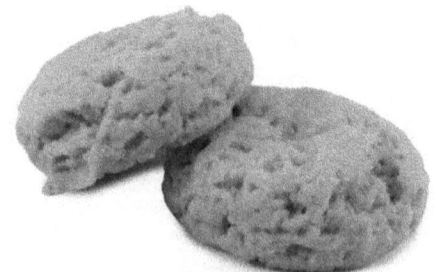

Today, tell yourself:
Appreciation spreads through my thoughts
and actions and flows into my world.

Cheesy Corn Muffins

Ingredients
1/3 (11 oz.) bag cheese puffs
1/3 (16 oz.) bag tortilla chips
1/3 (16 oz.) bag corn chips
1 sleeve Saltine crackers
3 pkgs. chili Ramen seasonings
1 large spread bowl
1 coffee mug
1/3 coffee mug hot water
1/3 (16 oz.) bottle squeeze cheese

Directions
Crush cheese puffs, all chips, and saltine crackers. Set cheese puffs aside for a moment. Combine chips, crackers, and 1 chili seasoning in a large spread bowl. In a coffee mug, add two seasonings to a 1/3 coffee mug of hot water and stir until all dissolve. Add half the cheese to the mug and stir well. Pour this mixture into the spread bowl and quickly stir. Add cheese puffs to this and stir once more. Cover the bowl and allow it to sit for 30 minutes. Once time is up, divide the mixture into 8-10 parts and form your muffins. Allow to sit for another 15 minutes. Top with the remaining cheese and eat it up.

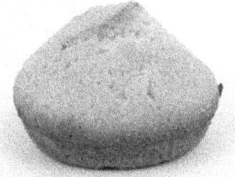

Today, tell yourself:
I have the power to create positive change in my life.

Troy Traylor

Chicken Biscuits

Ingredients

2 rolls snack crackers
2 pkgs. chicken Ramen seasoning

Directions

Quick, fast, and easy. Simply put all crackers in a clean, large chip bag. Add seasonings and shake the bag until all are coated. That's it, eat up.

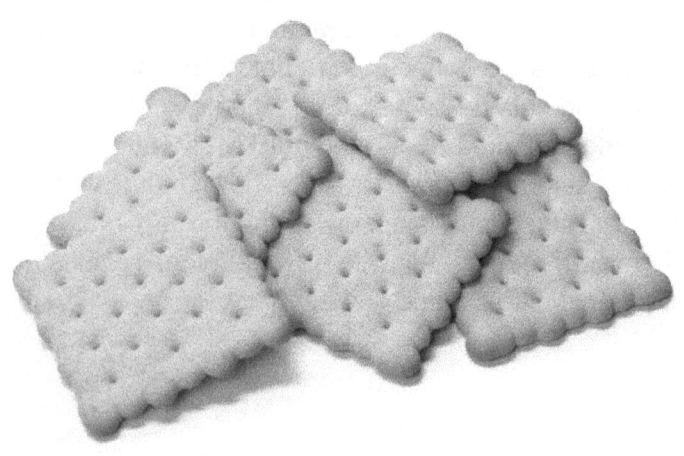

*Today, tell yourself:
This day is ripe with new
beginnings and fresh starts.*

Chicken Biscuits 2

Ingredients
2 rolls snack crackers
2 sleeves saltine crackers
1 large spread bowl
2 pkgs. chicken Ramen seasoning
1 pkg. vegetable Ramen seasoning
3 Tbsp. hot water
1 rice bag

Directions
Crush all crackers and place them in a spread bowl. Add seasoning packages and 2 tablespoons of water to this and knead well. You only want this mixture moist enough, so it all sticks together without breaking up. May need to add a few more drops of water for proper consistency. Divide this mixture into two equal parts and shape into your biscuits. Place both biscuits in your rice bag and set down in your hot pot for 1 ½ hours. Eat these with your favorite meal.

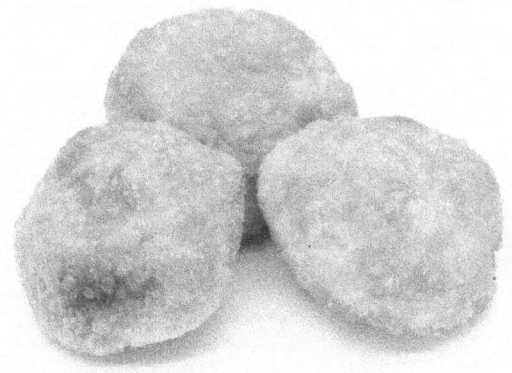

Today, tell yourself:
Joy is everywhere; I choose to see it.

Jalapeno Biscuits

Ingredients:

3 sleeves saltine crackers
2 rolls of snack crackers
¼ (16 oz.) bag tortilla chips
4 (1.3 oz.) jalapeno peppers
2 chili Ramen seasonings
2 Tbsp. hot sauce
1/3 coffee mug hot water
1 large spread bowl
1 rice bag

Directions

Crush all crackers and chips. Dice up jalapeno peppers. Put hot sauce and seasonings in a 1/3 coffee mug of hot water and stir until all is dissolved. Now, combine all these ingredients in a large spread bowl and mix thoroughly. Allow this bowl to sit, covered, for 30 minutes. Divide this mixture into 6 equal parts and shape your biscuits. Place two at a time in a clean rice bag and set down in your hot pot for 1-1 ½ hours to heat. Two hot pots work best, so you can eat faster.

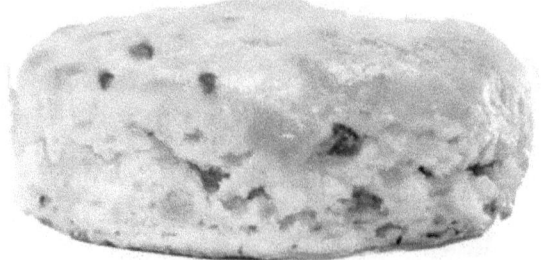

*Today, tell yourself:
This is my day, and I will use it
to be the best version of myself.*

Fine Dining Prison Cookbook 3

Jalapeno-Cheesy Corn Muffins

Ingredients
6 (1.3 oz.) jalapeno peppers
1/3 (11 oz.) bag cheese puffs
1/3 (16 oz.) bag tortilla chips
1/3 (16 oz.) bag corn chips
1 sleeve Saltine crackers
3 pkgs. chili Ramen seasonings
1 large spread bowl
1 coffee mug
1/3 coffee mug hot water
1/3 (16 oz.) bottle squeeze cheese

Directions
Dice up jalapeno peppers and crush cheese puffs. Set both aside for a moment. Now, crush all chips and crackers. Combine chips, crackers, 1 chili seasoning, and jalapeno peppers in a large spread bowl. In a coffee mug, add two seasoning packages with 1/3 coffee mug of hot water and stir until all dissolve. Add half the cheese to this mug and stir well. Pour this mixture into the spread bowl and quickly stir. Add cheese puffs to this and stir once more. Cover the bowl and allow it to sit for 30 minutes. Once time is up, divide the mixture into 8-10 parts and form your muffins. Allow to sit another 15 minutes. Top with remaining cheese and eat it up.

Today, tell yourself:
I see my life and the world in which
I live with grateful eyes.

Raisin Spice Biscuits

Ingredients
3 sleeves saltine crackers
1 roll snack crackers
1 good handful of raisins
1 Tbsp. cinnamon
2-1/2 Tbsp. water
1 large spread bowl
1 rice bag

Directions
Crush all crackers and combine all ingredients in a large spread bowl. Knead well and separate into 2-3 equal parts. Shape into biscuits and place in a rice bag. Set this bag in your hot pot and allow it to heat for 2 hours.

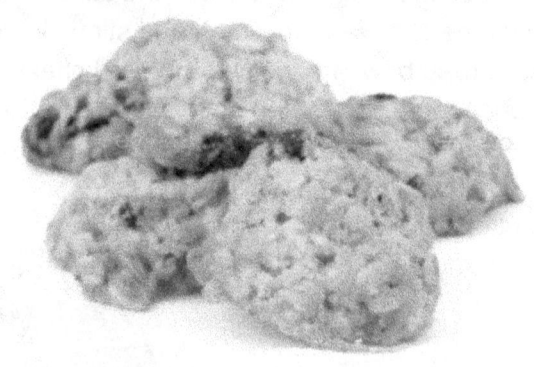

Today, tell yourself:
I can be happy whenever I want
no matter what my circumstances.

Food Facts

Fat

Fat is another one of the macronutrients. The past two food facts have covered the other partners: protein and carbohydrates. If you focus on the readings, then you will see I am trying to inform you about the necessary information first. One of the least understood things when it comes to structuring your diet is fat. So, does fat make you fat? Well, yes and no.

Different types of fat.

Dietary fat is defined as fat that comes from animals and plants and supplies our bodies as an essential macronutrient. There are two main types of dietary fat concern, trans-fat and saturated fat although there are others, such as monounsaturated, polyunsaturated, and polyunsaturated fats, like omega-3 fatty acids.

Trans-Fat

Also called trans-fatty acids or partially hydrogenated fats, trans fat is prevalent due to its low cost, convenience, and long shelf life. However, cheaper now does not mean cheaper in the long run. Heart disease and type-2 diabetes will certainly cost you more than that low-fat salad dressing. Trans fat raises your low-density lipoprotein (LDL) levels-which I guess we could call "bad" cholesterol. LDL increases the risk of cardiovascular disease, and HDL does the opposite.

Saturated fat

Saturated fats are called so because they consist of double-bonded molecules saturated with hydrogen. Don't know why that matters? You're not alone. Just consider that beef, poultry, cheese, and butter all naturally contain saturated fat and that it has been proven to reduce cardiovascular disease, as opposed to trans-fat, which increases it. But don't start thinking that you can just eat all the saturated fat you want without repercussions. Like trans-fat, saturated fat increases the level of bad cholesterol (that's LDL, by the way, for those paying attention) and may cause weight gain.

Omega-3

Omega-3 fatty acids are a type of unsaturated fatty acid found in a variety of foods that are often called "essential fatty acids" because, although your body doesn't produce them on its own, they are required for your body to function.

You can find Omega-3 fatty acids in a whole lot of food that is generally considered good for you, say fish and soy, just to name two. It helps decrease your appetite and has a positive effect on your energy levels and body temperature by increasing your body's secretion of a hormone called leptin. Looking for a solid source of Omega-3? Look no further than your nearest pack of tuna (one gram per 113g serving), salmon, or mackerel (each has two grams per 113g serving).

Consensus

Fat is a necessary part of your diet. Yes, overconsumption can lead to many health issues, but studies have shown that people who cut all fat from their diet and replace it with either only carbohydrates or protein gain more weight than those who make health-conscious choices when choosing which fats to intake and how frequently. Avoid trans-fats from processed foods and instead look at Omega-3 fatty acids from fish or supplements.

*Each life is lived differently
and today's day and age is tough,
start each day by appreciating everything.
but most importantly, appreciate your life
and yourself!*

Section 5:
Sides

Troy Traylor

Bold Stuffed Peppers

Ingredients
6 (1.3 oz.) jalapeno peppers
1 large spread bowl
1 (3.53 oz.) pkg. jalapeno tuna
3 (2 oz.) pkgs. cream cheese
½ Tbsp. hot sauce
1 Tbsp. no-salt seasoning
2 Matzo crackers (sub ½. Sleeve Saltine crackers)
1 rice bag

Directions
Cut the stems from the peppers and use the handle of a spoon to clean out the seeds in a large bowl. Set peppers aside. Add the jalapeno tuna, 2 packages of cream cheese, hot sauce, and no-salt seasoning to the bowl and mix well. Spoon this mixture back into the peppers. Crush your Matzo/saltine crackers. Using the last cream cheese, coat all peppers and roll in crackers to coat. Place these in a rice bag and set down in a hot pot to heat for 2 hours. Eat as a side or as is. Either way, you cannot go wrong.

Today, tell yourself:
Love is everywhere I am.

Pickle Boat

Ingredients
1 (9 oz.) pickle
1 pkg. meat of choice
1 (2 oz.) pkg. ranch dressing
1 tsp. onion powder
1 large spread bowl

Directions
Cut the pickle in half, lengthwise, and scrape out the seeds and some of the pulp to create your boat. Set this aside for a moment. Now, take your meat of choice, ranch dressing, and onion powder, and combine them all in a large spread bowl. Dice up seeds and pulp and add to the bowl. Stir well until all is thoroughly mixed. Now, spoon this mixture back into your boat and eat it up. A nice addition is topped with a few crushed cheese puffs. Simply delicious!

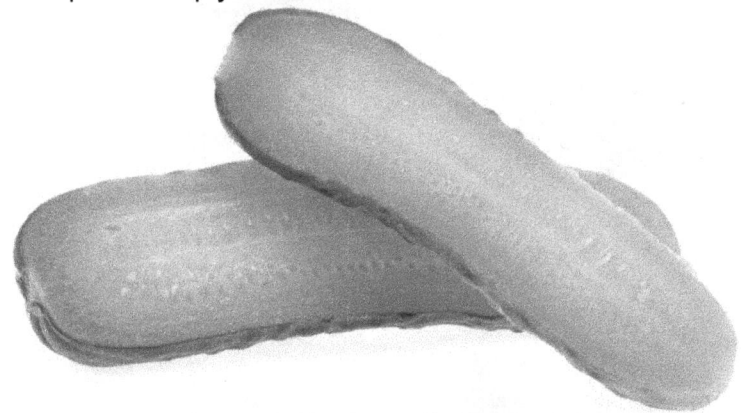

Today, tell yourself:
Life is a series of tiny miracles.
Today I choose to notice and be
thankful for all of them.

Ranch Style Bacon

Ingredients
1 (2.75 oz.) bag pork skins
1-2 (2 oz.) pkg(s) ranch dressing
3 Tbsp. water

Directions
Fastest recipe ever! Open a bag of pork skins, add 3 tablespoons of water, and shake until all the water is absorbed. Now top with ranch dressing and eat up. See how fast this one is? Can put it in a spread bowl or eat it right out of the bag. Either way, you'll enjoy this treat.

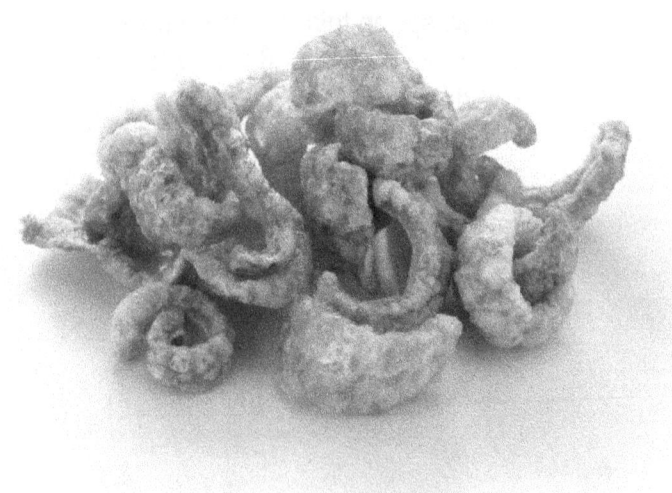

*Today, tell yourself:
Life is a journey, and I am growing
wiser, stronger, and braver by the day.*

Red Rice

Ingredients
1 (1.3 oz.) jalapeno pepper
1/4 (8 oz.) bag instant white rice
1-1/4 coffee mugs hot water
1 (2.75 oz.) bag pork skins

Directions
Dice jalapeno pepper. Combine all ingredients in a large spread bowl, stir, cover, and allow to cook for 10-12 minutes. Stir again after cooking time and eat up. I prefer to put pork skins on top after stirring the first time, so there is still a little crunch as I eat. But of course, this is your choice.

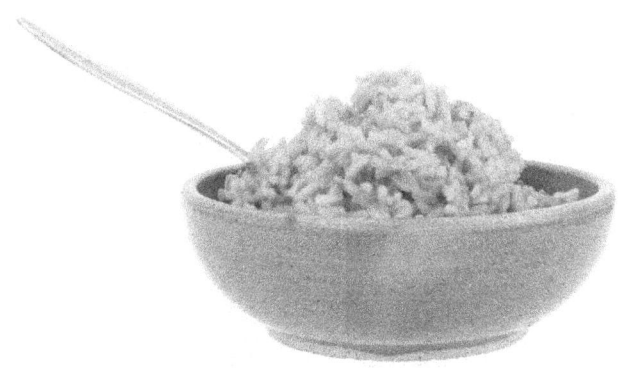

Today, tell yourself:
The past is over and gone
I create my future with the choices
I made today.

Sweet Fiery Rice

Ingredients
1 (8 oz.) bag instant white rice
2 coffee mugs with hot water (leave 4 Tbsp. for candy)
9 pcs. Fireball candies
6 pkgs. sweetener (sub 10 tsp. sugar)
1/2 (2 oz.) pkg. vanilla chike (protein powder)
1 heaping Tbsp. vanilla cappuccino
1 large spread bowl

Directions
Open the rice bag and pour in hot water. Wrap in a towel and allow to heat for 10-12 minutes. While waiting, crush fireball candies and put them in a coffee mug with 4 Tablespoons hot water. Stir until all dissolves. Once the rice is ready, combine all ingredients in a large spread bowl, stir well, and get ready for the best rice ever.

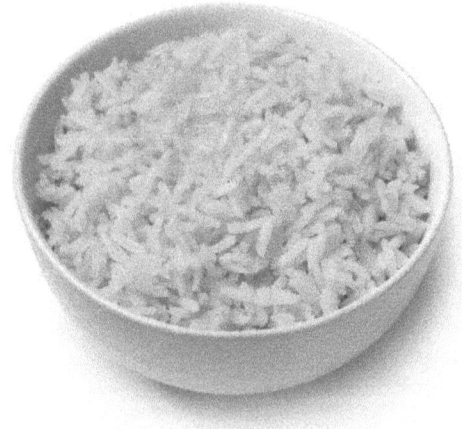

Today, tell yourself:
Every decision I make leads
me somewhere wonderful.

Fine Dining Prison Cookbook 3

Genius Granola Hacks

Sure, it's great on yogurt with fruit, but there are other innovative ways to enjoy this amazing breakfast classic that go beyond the bowl.

Freeze mini frozen parfait bars:
Stir 1 Tbsp. pure maple syrup into 1 cup of low-fat plain Greek yogurt. Divide among the wells of a 14-well ice cube tray. Sprinkle with ½ cup granola, then press a berry into each. Freeze until solid, at least 4 hours. Serves 14.

Add crunch to your pancakes:
Stir ½ cup granola into a batter made from 7 oz. (about 1 cup) whole wheat pancake mix. Coat a large non-stick skillet with cooking spray and heat over medium heat. For each pancake, sprinkle about 1 tsp. granola into the pan and top with a ¼ cup batter. Cook, flipping once halfway, until golden.
Serves 4: 2 each.

Whip up some bars:
Puree ½ cup pitted Medjool dates in a food processor, adding warm water 1 Tbsp. at a time to form a paste. Add 1 cup peanut butter and 2 ½ cups granola; pulse to combine. Press into an 8-inch baking dish lined with parchment paper. Refrigerate until firm, at least 1 hour. Cut into 12 bars.
Serves 12.

Top your salad:
Toss 2 cups of greens with 1 Tbsp. red-wine vinaigrette. Top with ¼ cup fresh berries and 2 Tbsp. each crumbled goat cheese and granola.
Serves 1.

Make sweet bread:
Melt ½ cup chocolate chips. Spread into a 6-inch square onto a parchment-lined baking sheet. Swirl in 1 Tbsp. jam and sprinkle with ½ cup granola. Refrigerate until set, about 15 minutes, then

53

break into 8 pieces.
Serves 8.

Toss it into a smoothie:
Blend ¾ cup low-fat milk, 1 cup frozen berries, ½ cup each granola and low-fat plain Greek yogurt, and 1 tsp. honey until smooth.
Serves 2: 1 cup each.

Bags to Buy

Here are some of the granolas that are most loved! Because serving sizes vary, these are converted to show values for 1/3 cup of each brand.

Bear Naked Fruit and Nut Granola:
180 Cal, 0mg sodium, 7g added sugar, 3g fiber, 4g protein
Featuring almonds, cranberries, raisins, and pecans, this mix has a satisfying amount of fiber and protein.

Nature's Path Love Crunch Dark Chocolate and Red Berries Granola:
173 Cal, 73mg sodium, 8g added sugar, 3g fiber, 3g protein
Satisfy your sweet tooth with this combo of dried strawberries and raspberries and decadent dark chocolate chunks.

Kind Healthy Grains Cinnamon Oat Granola with Flax Seeds:
110 Cal, 25mg sodium, 4g added sugar, 4g fiber, 3g protein
This fiber-packed granola contains 6 whole grains—oats, brown rice, buckwheat, millet, amaranth, quinoa, plus flaxseeds, and just enough cinnamon.

Buyers Guide

French Green Lentils:
Loaded with fiber and protein, French Green Lentils hold their shape when cooked, making them a good candidate for salads. You can find these in natural foods stores and specialty markets.

Creole Mustard:
Defined by its horseradish flavor, Creole mustard gets its signature spice from the brown seeds of Louisiana-grown mustard greens. You can find this at your local market with other mustards or online.

Creamed Honey:
Despite its appearance, creamed honey features just one ingredient: honey. This sweetener runs through a low-temperature process designed to control crystallization and keep it soft and spreadable. You can look for this with other kinds of honey at your local grocery store or online.

Torani Puremade Sauces:
Whether perking up your morning coffee or enhancing a treat in the evening, Torani Puremade Sauces can bring some flavor to each day. Kettle-crafted with no artificial ingredients or preservatives, Torani can be added to any beverage or dessert for deliciousness without compromise.

Two Helpful Tips

Make Time for Breakfast:
As the most important meal of the day, breakfast gets your mind and body going. Fueling your day with a healthy breakfast is sure to get you moving so you can take on each day your way!

8 Hours Every Night:
Sleep is the body's most important time to rest and reset. Studies show that getting eight hours of sleep every night can

help improve your health, concentration, and overall mood.

Food Facts

What's the Difference?
All white rice begins as brown rice. To increase the rice's shelf life and decrease its cooking time, brown rice undergoes a milling process that removes the bran, germ, and husk and leaves only the individual grain. A side effect of this process is that much of the rice's nutritional value is depleted. To combat this, the newly shorn white rice is "enriched" with nutrients and polished to make it look more palatable.

While both are high in carbs and low in calories and are generally considered a healthy choice, brown rice is a whole grain and thus can help lower your risk of stroke, Type 2 Diabetes, and heart disease. It can also assist you in keeping your cholesterol low.

Fiber
Brown rice provides one to three grams more fiber than white rice per 100 grams. Men under the age of 50 typically require 38 grams of fiber per day. Fiber helps you feel fuller faster, which can help you manage your weight, lower your cholesterol, reduce your risk of both heart disease and diabetes, aid in the relief of constipation, and nourish your gut bacteria.

Other Nutrients
White rice falls short of its whole-grain counterpart in several other nutritional areas. Brown is a good source of manganese, a mineral essential for energy production; selenium, which helps with immune function and thyroid hormone production and works with Vitamin E in protecting cells from cancer; and magnesium, another mineral necessary for a swath of vital functions, including muscle contraction and bone development. A half cup of brown rice can provide you with 11% of your daily recommended value of magnesium. White rice scores its one hit with folate, offering almost half your daily recommended amount in a one-cup serving. Folate gives your body a hand in making DNA and supports cell division, resulting in fewer birth defects.

Consensus

The food facts seem stacked against white rice. Despite its cleaner look, longer shelf, and faster prep time, it provides little of the nutritional content found in brown rice. And get this: where brown rice decreases your risk of Type 2 Diabetes by 32% when made a regular part of your diet, white rice is known to increase the risk factor by 17%.

Pro Tip

Don't know how to accurately measure your rice or other dry foods? If in prison, use the lid on your hot pot: it measures out exactly one dry cup. When cooking brown rice, allow for more prep time. Also, the best practice is to rinse the rice in cold water before cooking to remove any extra starch and dust.

Pinto Beans, Black Eye Beans, & Vegetable Beans

Pinto Beans
Serving Size: ¼ cup
Calories per serving: 80 (% Daily Value)
Total Fat 0.5g
Trans Fat 0g
Cholesterol 0mg
Sodium 140 mg (6%)
Total Carbohydrates 22g (8%)
Dietary Fiber 11g (41%)
Sugars 6g
Protein 7g

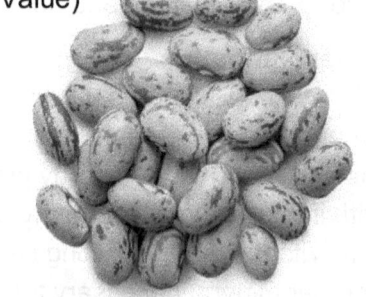

*Percent Daily Values are based on a 2,000-calorie diet.

Pinto beans are extremely nutritious. They're an excellent source of protein, fiber, vitamins, and minerals. These nutrients may provide several benefits, including improved blood sugar control and heart health. They are also rich in various antioxidants. This may help lower your risk of chronic disease. The soluble fiber found in beans slows down your digestion and has been proven to lower cholesterol, keeping your heart healthy and great for blood glucose control. Eating pinto beans can also reduce the rise in blood sugar that happens after eating a meal.

Black Eye Beans

Serving Size: 1/3 cup
Calories per serving: 100(% Daily Value)
Total Fat 0g
Saturated Fat 0g
Trans Fat 0g
Cholesterol 0mg
Sodium 15mg (1%)
Total Carbohydrates 23g (8%)
Dietary Fiber 10g (36%)
Sugars 1g
Protein 9g

*Percent Daily Values are based on a 2,000-calorie diet.

Black-eyed beans or black-eyed peas are rich in fiber and protein, which makes them an excellent energy source. They may help support weight loss, improve heart health, and promote digestive health. Fiber helps keep you regular and seems to protect against heart disease, high cholesterol, high blood pressure, and digestive illness.

Vegetarian Beans

Serving Size: ½ cup
Calories per serving: 120 (% Daily Value)
Total Fat 0g
Saturated Fat 0g
Trans Fat 0g

Cholesterol 0mg
Sodium 140mg (6%)
Dietary Fiber 5g (18%)
Sugars 6g
Protein 7g

* Percent Daily Values are based on a 2,000-calorie diet.

What's the difference between vegetarian beans and regular beans? Vegetarian beans are beans that are made without the addition of meat, poultry, fish, or meat flavorings. All beans, by their very definition, are vegetarian. Overall, legume consumption has been linked to heart health, appetite control, and weight management, as well as blood sugar regulation. Also, legumes appear to lower total LDL cholesterol as well as lower blood pressure.

Food Facts

Carbohydrates: Simple vs. Complex

What is a carbohydrate?
Carbohydrates – or carbs – are molecules composed of oxygen, hydrogen, and carbon, and they are one of three macronutrients– the other two being fat and protein. The terms simple and complex are in reference to their molecular structure, and they can make a big difference.

There are three different types of carbohydrates: fiber and starches, which are complex, and sugars, which are simple. While most people think of pasta when they hear "carbs," the truth is you can find them in a variety of foods. Many foods contain both.

Complex
Complex carbs have longer molecular chains that take longer to break down and thus digest more efficiently. This gives you longer-lasting energy than simple carbs provide. They are high in nutrients and fiber, which aids in the digestion process. Fiber also helps one feel fuller, aiding in weight loss. People with Type 2 Diabetes should look to include more complex carbs in their diet to help manage sugar spikes. Here are some examples of foods that contain large amounts of complex carbs:

> Whole wheat bread
> Rice
> Oats
> Cereal
> Whole Grains
> Beans
> Fiber-rich fruit and vegetables

Simple Carbs
Simple carbs are digested rapidly and disperse energy into the bloodstream immediately. That may sound good, but following

that burst, you can be sure to expect a fatigue-filled crash. Some simple carbs occur naturally in things like milk, but most simple carbs are additives.

There are numerous studies showing that regular consumption of simple-sometimes, also called refined carbs-is associated with Type 3 Diabetes, obesity, and numerous other chronic illnesses. Here are some examples of foods that contain high amounts of simple carbs and should thus be avoided if you are trying to maintain a healthy diet.

> Packaged cookies
> Soda
> Fruit juice concentrate
> Breakfast cereal
> Pastries

Consensus
Stay away from simple carbs as much as you can. There are some foods in which simple carbs occur naturally and can be a part of a healthy diet, but the majority are just no good. Simple carbs are sometimes called "empty" because they lack so many essential nutrients. Complex carbs assist you in managing your energy and weight and help you keep a better diet overall because so many foods that are healthy for other reasons contain them. Many "low-carb" diets tend to promote the idea that carbohydrates contribute to obesity. This is simply not true. Carbs are good for you, just to make sure you pay attention and keep them complex.

*The golden key in life is acceptance.
Accept yourself and accept others,
and always remember that you can
change the way you feel by changing
the way you think.*

Section 6:
Meals of All Kinds

Troy Traylor

Baltimore's Bagin' Burrito

Ingredients
1 (16 oz.) bag corn chips
3 (3 oz.) chili Ramen noodles
1 large chip bag
1-3/4 coffee mugs hot water
3 (3.53 oz.) pkgs. jalapeño tuna
1 large spread bowl
squeeze cheese to taste
1 (2 oz.) pkg. ranch dressing
hot sauce to taste

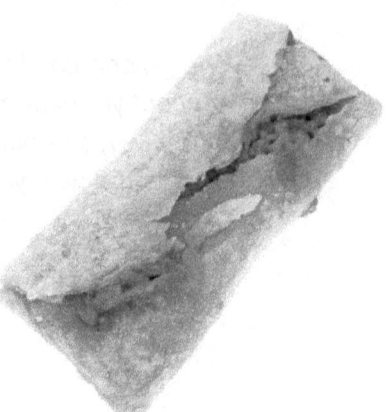

Directions
Crush corn chips and Ramen noodles. Put these in a large chip bag with seasonings. Add hot water to the bag and knead until the water is absorbed. Flatten out in the chip bag, a little thicker than a pizza crust. Wrap the bag in a towel for 10-12 minutes. While waiting, combine jalapeno tuna and cream cheese in a large spread bowl and mix well. Remove pretzels from your party mix and set them aside. Crush this party mix and set it aside as well. Once cooking time is up, unwrap the bag and cut it open. Top with tuna mixture. Spread evenly, about 1 inch from each end. Now cover with crushed party mix and squeeze cheese. Carefully roll this up to shape a burrito. Now cover with ranch dressing and hot sauce. Better be hungry for this one.

*Today, tell yourself:
I trust that everything is happening
now, it is happening for my benefit.*

Cheesy Vegan Pasta

Ingredients
2 (3 oz.) vegetable Ramen noodles
1 large spread bowl
2 coffee mugs refried beans
4 coffee mugs hot water
1/3 (16 oz.) bottle squeeze cheese
2 (2 oz.) pkgs. ranch dressing

Directions
Crush Ramen and place it in a spread bowl. Add your refried beans and hot water to the bowl, stir, and cover for 10 minutes. Pour off any remaining water once cooking time is up. Add vegetable seasoning and cheese, stir well, and top with ranch.

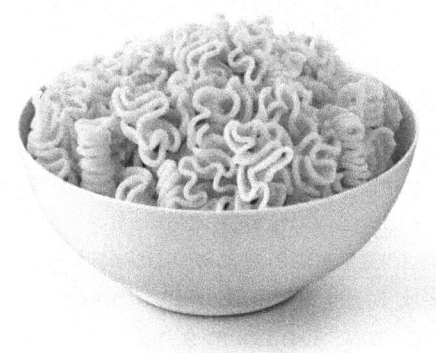

*Today, tell yourself:
I am much kinder,
a happier version of myself,
and I've only just begun.*

Troy Traylor

Chicken-Chili Taquitos

Ingredients
4 Tbsp. salsa
1 pkg. chicken Ramen seasoning
1 pkg. spicy vegetable Ramen seasoning
½ tsp. onion powder
¼ tsp. garlic powder
½ tsp. no-salt seasoning
½ (8 oz.) bag instant white rice
2 coffee mugs hot water
2 (1.3 oz) jalapeno peppers
1/3 (8 oz.) bag Shabang chips
1 large spread bowl
1 (8 oz.) pkg. chicken chili
¼ (16 oz.) bottle squeeze cheese
1 (10 oz.) pkg. flour tortillas

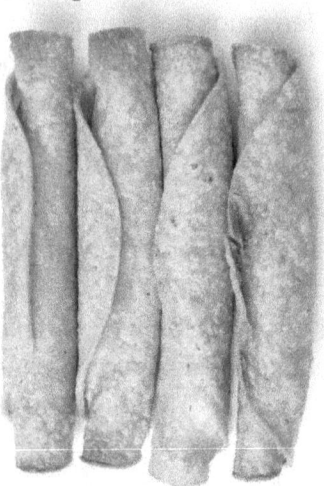

Directions
Add salsa and all seasonings to the rice bag, along with 2 coffee mugs of hot water. Shake until all is mixed and wrap in a towel for 10 minutes. While waiting, dice jalapeno peppers, crush chips, and combine these in a large spread bowl. Set flour tortillas aside, combine the remaining ingredients in this bowl, and mix well. Once the rice is ready, add the contents of the bag to the bowl and mix well again. Now, spoon 3 good Tablespoons of mixture onto flour tortillas, tuck ends, and roll up. Place 4 taquitos into the rice bag and set in a hot pot to heat for 45 minutes. Repeat until all is gone. It should make 12 nice taquitos.

Today, tell yourself:
I know myself; I trust myself,
and I can be myself.

Chickles

Ingredients
2 (9 oz.) pickles
1 (2 oz.) bag small chips of choice
2 large chip bags
1 (7 oz.) pkg. chicken chunks
1 tsp. garlic powder

Directions
Cut pickles in half lengthwise and clean out seeds and some pulp. Drain chicken chunks and crush chips. Combine chicken chunks, chips, and garlic in a large chip bag and thoroughly mix. Double bag and set down in a hot pot to heat for 45 minutes. Spoon back into the pickle halves and eat them up. Top with a little ranch if desired.

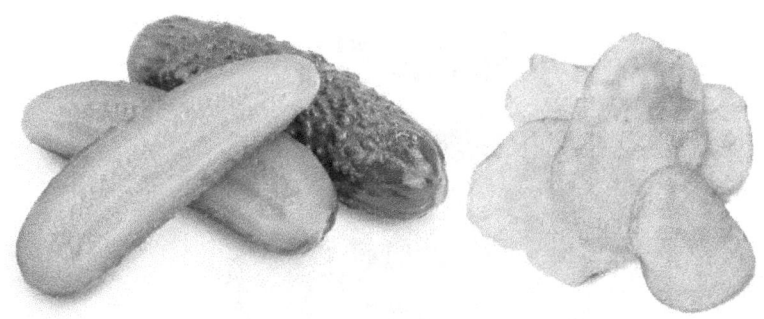

Today, tell yourself:
This is my moment. Every
step and misstep have led me here.

Chili Cheese Soup

Ingredients
2 (3 oz.) chili Ramen noodles
3 coffee mugs hot water
1 large spread bowl
1 (2.75 oz.) bag pork skins
1 coffee mug crushed party mix (remove pretzels)
2 Tbsp. hot sauce
6 Tbsp. squeeze cheese

Directions
Prepare Ramen with seasonings in hot water in a large bowl. Do not drain. Now combine all remaining ingredients, mix well, cover for 10 minutes, and enjoy. It's just a simple way to get through any day.

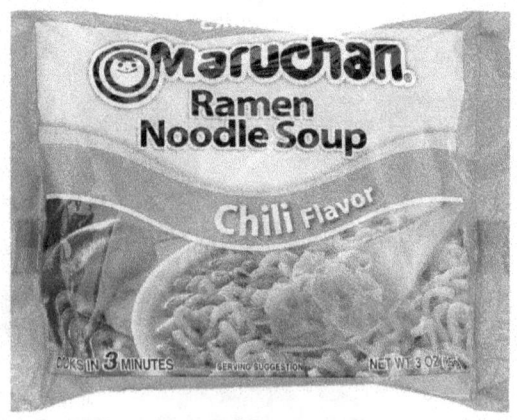

*Today, tell yourself:
No matter what happens
I am always all right.*

Chili Cheese Soupy Soup

Ingredients
2 (3 oz.) chili Ramen noodles
3 pkgs. chili Ramen noodle seasoning
½ Tbsp. garlic powder
1 Tbsp. onion powder
7 Tbsp. kosher chili beans
5 heaping Tbsp. instant white rice
½ (16 oz.) bottle squeeze cheese
1 large spread bowl
1 (1.3 oz.) jalapeno pepper
½ (9 oz.) pickle
3 coffee mugs hot water
¼ (8 oz.) bag Shabang chips

Directions
Split the Ramen in half, then quarter each half. You'll have 16 pieces. Combine Ramen, all seasonings, kosher beans, and rice, and squeeze cheese together in a large bowl. Dice up pepper and pickle and add to bowl with 3 coffee mugs of hot water. Stir and cover for 10-12 minutes. Crush Shabang chips and top.

*Today, tell yourself:
I have a well-balanced point
of view, I can find the
good in everything.*

Troy Traylor

Chinese Anyone

Ingredients
2 (3 oz.) spicy vegetable Ramen noodles
3 coffee mugs hot water
1 large spread bowl
1 (3.53 oz.) pkg jalapeno tuna
1/3 (2.75 oz.) bag pork skins
1 (2 oz.) pkg. energizer mix
1 Tbsp. hot sauce
1 tsp. garlic powder
5 Tbsp. BBQ sauce

Directions
Lightly crush Ramen noodles and prepare without seasoning packets, in 3 coffee mugs of hot water, in a large spread bowl. Cover and allow to sit for 8 minutes. Do not drain excess water. Now, set the BBQ sauce aside and add the seasoning packets and remaining ingredients. Stir well, cover, and allow to set for an additional 5 minutes. Top with BBQ sauce and dig in. Thank you very much.

Today, tell yourself:
I give myself permission
to do what makes me happy.

Chinese Chicken

Ingredients
1 (7 oz.) pkg. chicken chunks
1 (3 oz.) chicken Ramen noodles
1 (.14 oz.) pkg. orange electrolytes
2 pkgs. sweetener (sub 4 tsp. sugar)
1 (8 oz.) bag instant white rice
3 coffee mugs hot water
1 (2.75 oz.) bag pork skins
1 large spread bowl
1/3 (18 oz.) bottle BBQ sauce
1 (2 oz.) pkg. ranch dressing
2 hot pots work best for this recipe

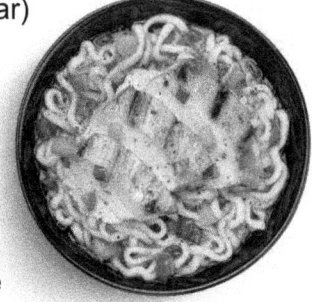

Directions
Rinse off the chicken chunks package and set it down in a hot pot to heat. While waiting for chicken to heat, crush Ramen noodles. Add Ramen noodles, seasoning package, electrolytes, and sweeteners to the rice bag, with enough hot water to cover all, about 1 inch over the top. Seal the bag, wrap it in a towel, and let sit for 10-12 minutes. While waiting, crush half the bag of pork skins and leave the other half whole. Set crushed pork skins aside. Use a spread bowl and combine BBQ sauce and whole pork skins. Stir around and allow these to soak. Once all is hot/prepped, put the rice mixture in a separate spread bowl and top with chicken chunks and crushed pork skins. Mix well. Top off with soaked pork skins and ranch dressing. Grab a cold drink and enjoy.

Today, tell yourself:
"I am sincerely grateful to those who I am,
where I am, and what I have."

Cowboy Tacos

Ingredients
1 (5 oz.) summer sausage
1 (4 oz.) bag turkey/chicken bites
½ Tbsp. garlic powder
1 Tbsp. onion powder
½ coffee mug hot water
1 rice bag
½ coffee mug refried beans
2 Tbsp. hot sauce of choice
1/3 (8 oz.) bag Shabang chips
6 flour tortillas
6 Tbsp. salsa/picante sauce

Directions
Dice up summer sausage and turkey/chicken bites. Combine meat, seasonings, and hot water in a rice bag and shake a bit. Set the bag down in a hot pot to heat for 30 minutes. After this cook-time, add refried beans, hot sauce, and whole chips to this bag and set it back down in the hot pot for an additional 30 minutes. Stir occasionally. Now spoon mixtures onto the flour tortillas, roll up and top with salsa/picante sauce. One meal to enjoy!

> Today, tell yourself:
> I am letting clarity, appreciation,
> and confidence leads the way.

Creamy Chicken for Two

Ingredients
2 (3 oz.) chicken Ramen noodles
3 coffee mugs hot water
2 large spread bowls
3 (2 oz.) pkgs. cream cheese
2 Tbsp. onion powder
1 Tbsp. garlic powder
black pepper to taste
½ coffee mug instant milk
3 Tbsp. squeeze cheese
1 hot pot insert cup
1 (7 oz.) pkg. chicken chunks

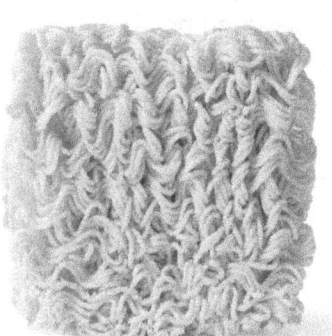

Directions
Leave Ramen noodles whole, and in bowl #1, combine Ramen, seasonings, and hot water in a large spread bowl. Cover and allow to cook for 10 minutes. Drain excess water (broth) into an insert cup and set aside. Now, in bowl #2, combine cream cheese, onion powder, garlic powder, black pepper, instant milk, and squeeze cheese. Whip until thoroughly mixed. Carefully pour in broth and stir until you reach your desired consistency. If there is no broth, then add a little water and a chicken seasoning package. Pour this into an insert cup and set it down in a hot pot to heat for 30 minutes. Stir occasionally. Heat chicken chunks in their package in a second hot pot. Once all cooking time is up, pour chicken chunks into bowl #1. Stir and top with broth mixture. Stir well and enjoy one amazing meal.

Today, tell yourself:
Every day I can create new habits
that will get me closer to where
and who I want to be.

Troy Traylor

EZ Cheezy Tuna Delight

Ingredients
1 (9 oz.) bag pasta shells
1 large spread bowl
2-1/2 coffee mugs hot water
¼ (4 oz.) bag instant milk
1/3 (16 oz.) bottle squeeze cheese
1-1/2 tsp. garlic powder
3 (3.53 oz.) pkgs. jalapeno tuna
1 (4 oz.) pkg. turkey bites

Directions
Carefully cook pasta shells in two cups hot water in a large spread bowl. These cook fast, so I suggest 4-5 minutes. Drain excess water. In your coffee mug, dissolve instant milk with water. Add milk mixture, squeeze cheese, and garlic powder into bowl, and stir well. Cover the bowl and allow to sit for 10 minutes. While waiting drain tuna packages, and dice turkey bites. Once the wait time is up, add these to the bowl and stir well. Better invite an associate for this one.

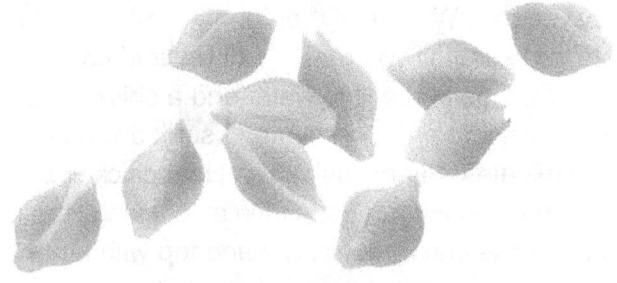

Today, tell yourself:
Yesterday is history, and tomorrow
is a mystery, Today is all I have
and I am grateful.

Fine Dining Prison Cookbook 3

Fabulous Fish Balls

Ingredients
1 (8 oz) bag jalapeno chips
2 (2.75 oz.) bags pork skins
1 (3.5 oz.) pkgs. mackerel
1 (2 oz.) pkg. ranch dressing
1 (2 oz.) pkg. cream cheese
3 Tbsp. onion powder
1 Tbsp. garlic powder
2 Tbsp. no-salt seasoning
4 Tbsp. BBQ sauce

Directions
Crush jalapeno chips and pork skins in their bags. Drain the fish package. Set one bag of pork skins aside, combine all remaining ingredients in the jalapeno chips bag, and mix thoroughly. Once thoroughly mixed, roll the mixture into your preferred size balls. Once all are rolled, use the remaining bag of pork skins to coat each one. Allow these to sit for 30 minutes to set up and dig in; it's time to eat.

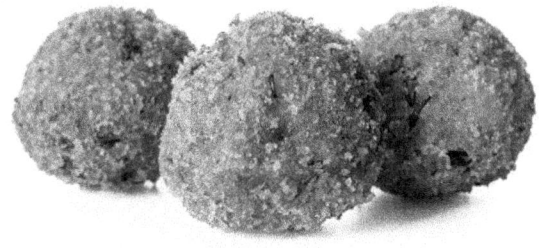

Today, tell yourself:
Today is the very first day
to the rest of my life.

Troy Traylor

Four Cheese Potato Meat Delight

Ingredients
1 (5 oz.) summer sausage
1 (3 oz.) pkg. Spam
1 (1.3 oz) jalapeno pepper
2 large spread bowls
1 chili Ramen seasoning
½ (2.75 oz.) bag pork skins
¼ (15 oz.) bag refried beans
4-1/2 coffee mugs hot water
¼ (10 oz.) bag four cheese instant potatoes
2 (2 oz.) pkgs. ranch dressing

Directions
Dice summer sausage, Spam, and jalapeno pepper and put all in a large spread bowl. Now add seasoning and lightly crushed pork skins to this, along with refried beans and 2 coffee mugs of hot water. Quickly stir and cover. Allow it to sit for 15 minutes. In a separate bowl, combine your instant potatoes and hot water. Whip until thick and creamy. Once the bean mixture is done, pour it over potatoes and top with ranch dressing. Great meal for a hungry man.

Today, tell yourself:
My life is getting better
because I am getting better.

Freaked Out Fluffy Potatoes

Ingredients
1 (8 oz.) bag jalapeno chips
1 (11.25 oz) pkg. chili no beans
2 large spread bowls
¼ (10 oz.) bag instant potatoes (any flavor)
1 Tbsp. garlic powder
1 (4 oz.) pkg. turkey/chicken bites
2 (2 oz.) pkgs. ranch dressing
2 (1.3 oz.) jalapeno peppers

Directions
Crush chips in the bag and add chili, no beans to this. Mix well and double bag. Set this down in a hot pot to heat for 1 hour. Right before cooking time is up, using a large spread bowl, combine instant potatoes, garlic powder, and hot water. Stir well. May need to add a little water to reach your desired texture. Cover the bowl for 3 minutes. Split the potatoes between 2 separate bowls. Remove the mixture from the hot pot and pour ½ into one bowl and ½ into the other. Don't stir. Pour cheese over the top and split the turkey bites/chicken bites between these two bowls. Top with one ranch in each bowl. Dice peppers and cover bowls to finish off. You can dice your turkey/chicken bites if you desire. I personally leave them whole.

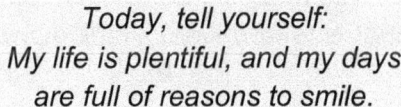

Today, tell yourself:
My life is plentiful, and my days
are full of reasons to smile.

Troy Traylor

Garbage Can Rice

Ingredients
½ (8 oz.) bag instant white rice
1 good shot squeeze cheese
4 Tbsp. no-salt seasoning
1 tsp. black pepper
1 pkg. spicy vegetable Ramen seasoning
2 coffee mugs hot water
1 large spread bowl

Directions
Combine all ingredients in a large spread bowl, stir well, tightly cover, and allow to heat for 15 minutes. It tastes far better than it sounds.

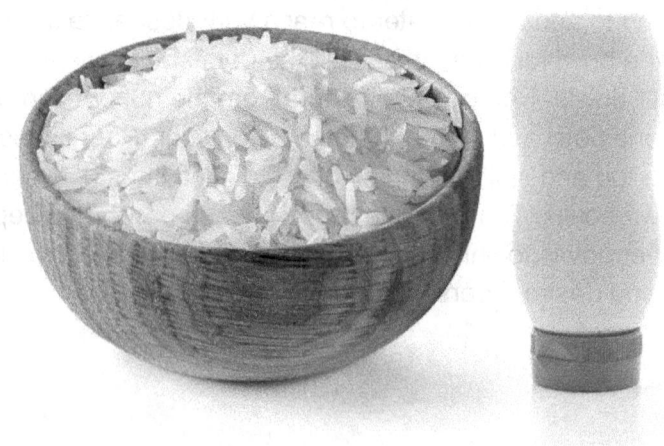

*Today, tell yourself:
I invite appreciation to stay; fear
doubt, and worry about falling away.*

Fine Dining Prison Cookbook 3

Get-Er-Done-Ramen

Ingredients
1 (3 oz.) Ramen noodles (any flavor)
1 large spread bowl
1-1/2 coffee mugs hot water
3 Tbsp. BBQ sauce
10 pork skins (leave whole)
1 good shot squeeze cheese

Directions
Crush Ramen noodles and place them in a large bowl. Add all remaining ingredients, stir well, cover tightly, and allow to heat for 6-8 minutes. That's it. Get it done and eat up.

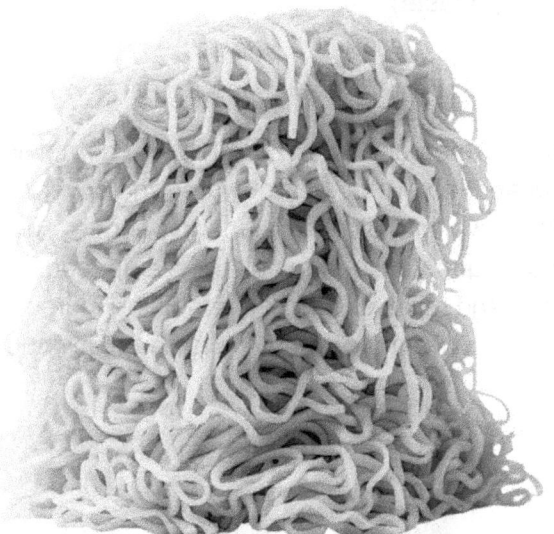

*Today, tell yourself:
I am grateful for every
challenging moment,
for they are my teachers.*

Gluten-Free Shindig

Ingredients
1/3 (8 oz.) bag instant rice
1 coffee mug refried beans
½ (2.75) bag pork skins (leave whole)
1 coffee mug corn chips (lightly crushed)
1 large spread bowl
4 coffee mugs water
2 (1.3 oz.) jalapeno peppers
2 (3.5 oz.) pkgs. mackerel
¼ (18 oz.) bottle BBQ sauce
squeeze cheese (to taste)
2 Tbsp. hot sauce
no salt seasoning (to taste)
onion powder (to taste)

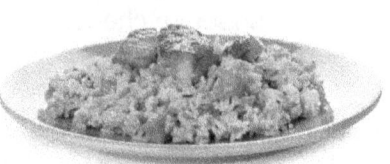

Directions
Combine rice, refried beans, pork skins, and corn chips in a spread bowl and mix well. Add hot water and cover for 10 minutes. While waiting, dice up jalapeno peppers and drain the mackerel packages. Once the cook time is up, add the peppers and mackerel and mix well. Add all remaining ingredients and mix thoroughly. Have a nice meal while you enjoy your favorite programs.

> *Today, tell yourself:*
> *I am at ease with my strengths*
> *and weaknesses, my successes*
> *and my challenges.*

Hungry Man's Belt-Busting Tacos

Ingredients

1 (8 oz.) bag instant white rice
3 coffee mugs hot water
1 (2.75 oz.) bag pork skins
1 (11 oz.) bag party mix (remove pretzels)
1 (3 oz.) bag nacho chips
1 (7 oz.) pkg. chicken chunks
1 (3 oz.) pkg. Spam
1 (4 oz.) pkg. turkey/chicken bites
3 (1.3 oz.) jalapeno peppers
1 large trash bag
1 pkg. spicy vegetable Ramen seasoning
1 pkg. chicken Ramen seasoning
1 Tbsp. garlic powder
2 Tbsp. onion powder
½ (16 oz.) bottle squeeze cheese
1 (12 oz.) V-8 juice
3 large spread bowls
3 (2 oz.) pkgs. cream cheese
1 (8 oz.) bottle of salsa

Directions

Cook rice in its bag, using 3 coffee mugs hot water. Wrap in a towel while cooking for 10-12 minutes. While waiting, crush up pork skins, all chips, and dice up all meats and jalapeno peppers. Now set the cream cheese and salsa aside, and using the large trash bags, combine the remaining ingredients and carefully knead well. Take your time to be sure all is equally mixed. Divide this mixture between the three spread bowls. Make a little crater in the center of each bowl. Once the rice is ready, split the rice between the bowls and top with the cream cheese and salsa. One amazing meal to share with a close associate.

Today, tell yourself:
I will use this day to find moments
of pleasure. And meaning in all I do.

Meaty Shells and Cheese

Ingredients
1 (9 oz.) bag pasta shells
1 coffee mug hot water
1 large spread bowl
1 (5 oz.) summer sausage
2 (2 oz.) pkgs. cream cheese
1/3 (16 oz.) bottle squeeze cheese
½ (8 oz.) bag tater skins

Directions
Prepare pasta shells in hot water in a large bowl. Drain water. Dice summer sausage or any meat product into smaller pieces. Set tater skins aside, combine all remaining ingredients, and mix well. Now, crush tater skins and cover the top of your creation.

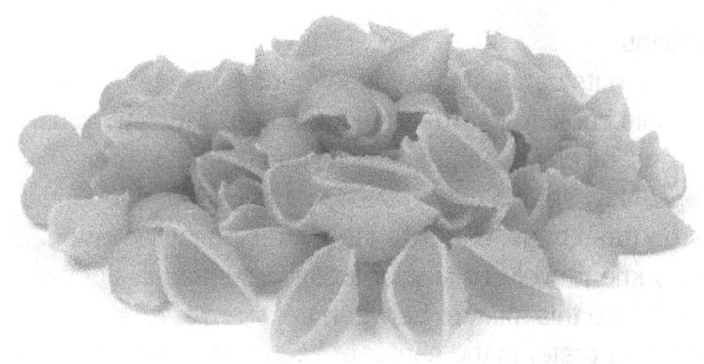

*Today, tell yourself:
Doors of opportunity are all around me, just waiting to be opened.*

Pork Skin-Tuna Delight

Ingredients
½ (2.75 oz.) bag pork skins
1 coffee mug refried beans
1-1/2 coffee mugs hot water
1 large spread bowl
1 (3.53 oz.) pkg. jalapeno tuna
1 (2 oz.) pkg. ranch dressing
1 good shot squeeze cheese

Directions
Combine pork skins, refried beans, and hot water in a large spread bowl, cover, and allow to cook for 10 minutes. Stir well and top with remaining ingredients.

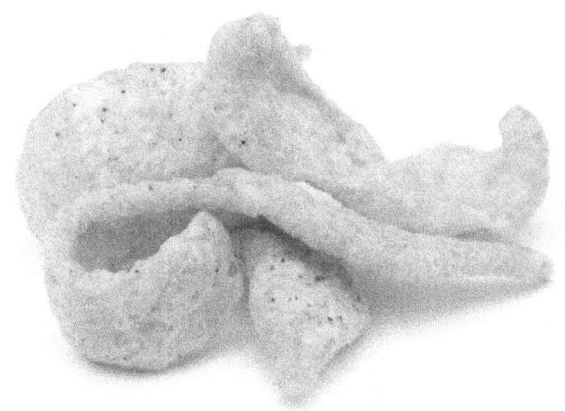

Today, tell yourself:
My problems and challenges are
nothing but a blessing in disguise.

Powerball Oatmeal Express

Ingredients
3 pkgs. instant oatmeal (any flavor)
1 (2 oz.) pkg. vanilla chike (protein powder)
1 large spread bowl
4 Tbsp hot water
1 large spread bowl

Directions
Combine oatmeal, chike, and cream cheese in a large spread bowl. Knead until thoroughly mixed. It will be very stiff. Add 4 Tablespoons hot water and knead again. Cover and allow to sit for 5 minutes. Roll the mixture into 8 balls and enjoy after a hard workout.

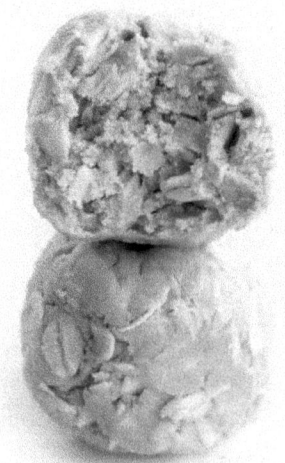

Today, tell yourself:
I will not focus on what I lack,
I will only focus on what I have.

Prison Pazole

Ingredients
½ (2.75 oz.) bag pork skins
1 (2 oz.) bag salted peanuts
2 Tbsp. no-salt seasoning
½ (8 oz.) bag instant white rice
2 coffee mugs hot water
2 large chip bags
1 large spread bowl

Directions
Combine all ingredients in a large chip bag. Mix well, double bag, and sit bag in a hot pot to heat for 2 hours. Pour it into a bowl and enjoy it with a nice cold drink.

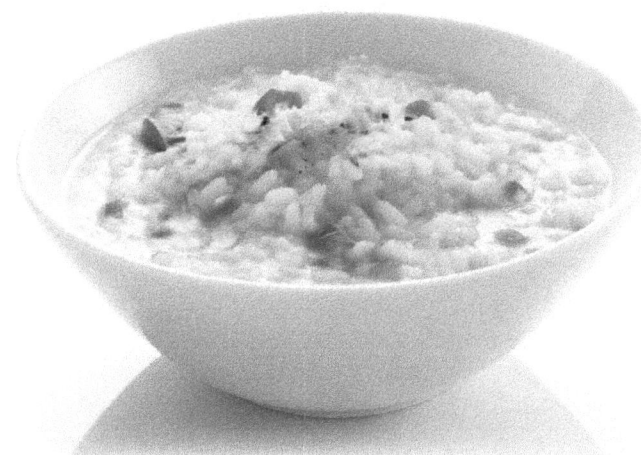

*Today, tell yourself:
I will leave behind old habits
and invite in new perspectives and fresh
ideas into my world.*

Salmon Cold Wraps

Ingredients
2 (5 oz.) pkgs. salmon
2 (2 oz.) pkgs. ranch dressing
2 (2 oz.) pkgs. energizer mix
1 tsp. no-salt seasoning
4 flour tortillas
2 large chip bags

Directions
Combine the first 4 ingredients together, mix well, and roll up into tortillas. Place all 4 in a large chip bag or double bag and set down in a hot pot to heat for one hour. This is a quick and healthy meal.

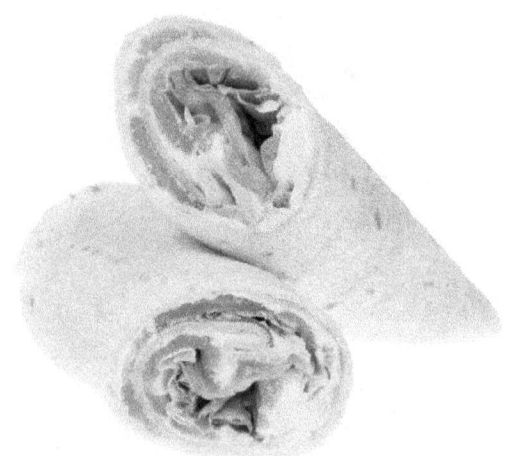

Today, tell yourself:
I choose to see my mistakes
as an experience to learn from.

Someone Say Queso

Ingredients
½ (9 oz.) pickle (diced)
1 (8 oz.) pkg. chicken chili
½ pkg. chili Ramen seasoning
½ (8 oz.) bottle salsa
½ (16 oz.) bottle squeeze cheese
3 handfuls tortilla chips
1 rice bag
1 large spread bowl

Directions
Combine the first 6 ingredients and put all in a rice bag. Set the bag in a hot pot to heat for 2 hours. Pour into your bowl and enjoy with saltine crackers. Nice meal.

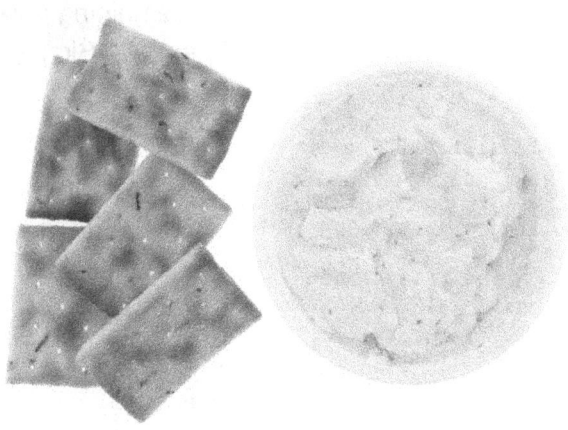

Today, tell yourself:
My heart is open, my mind
is at peace, and all is well.

Troy Traylor

Spicy Rice

Ingredients
2 (.14 oz.) pkg. orange electrolytes
1 (5.53 oz.) pkg. jalapeño tuna
½ (9 oz.) pickle
1 large spread bowl
1 (2.75 oz.) bag pork skins
2 (2 oz.) pkgs. ranch dressing
1 (2 oz.) bag salted peanuts

Directions
Add electrolytes to the rice bag along with hot water and jalapeno tuna. Stir, seal, and wrap in a towel to heat for 10-12 minutes. While waiting, dice up the pickle. When cooking time is up, add the rice mixture to a large bowl. Lightly crush pork skins. Add pickles, ½ bag pork skins, and one ranch dressing to the bowl and mix well. Top the dish off with remaining pork skins, additional ranch dressing, and salted peanuts. Simply delicious.

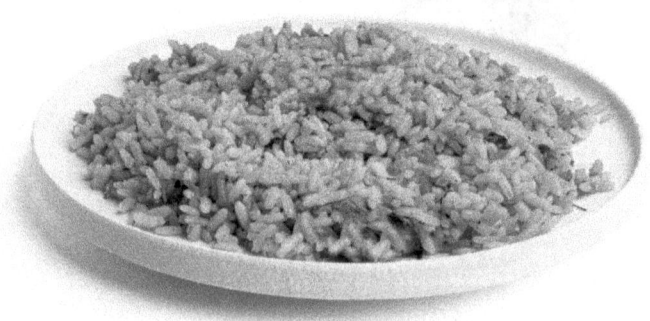

Today, tell yourself:
I have everything I need to
be happy and feel complete.

Stuffed Fish Balls

Ingredients
½ (8 oz.) bag Shabang chips
½ (8 oz.) bag jalapeno chips
1 (2.75 oz.) bag pork skins
1 (3.53 oz.) pkg. jalapeno tuna
1 (3.5 oz.) pkg. mackerel
4 Tbsp hot water
½ Tbsp. garlic powder
½ Tbsp. onion powder
1 (4 oz.) tub Gouda cheese (sub 1/3 bottle squeeze cheese)
1 (2 oz.) pkg. ranch dressing
hot sauce to taste
12 Tbsp. BBQ sauce
1 rice bag

Directions
Combine chips and pork skins in one bag and crush all. Do not drain fish packages. Add these packages to a chip bag, along with water and seasonings. Knead this mixture until all is combined. Flatten out the mixture in this chip bag and cut it open. You really want this just moist enough so that it all sticks together. May need to add another spoonful of water. Allow the mixture to sit for 15 minutes. Now, take a cheese bottle lid and cut 24 circles into the mixture. On top of 12 of the circles, put a dollop of Gouda or squeeze cheese. Put the remaining 12 circles on top of these and pinch all the way around each one to seal. Place 6 of these in a rice bag and set the bag down in a hot pot to heat for 45 minutes. Once done, top each one with ranch dressing, hot sauce, and BBQ sauce. It is a great meal served with buttered rice and refried beans. Repeat cooking directions for the remaining 6 fish balls.

*Today, tell yourself: to be grateful because
I love the way it makes me feel.*

Stuffed Pork

Ingredients
2 (1.3 oz.) jalapeno peppers
1 (2.75 oz.) bag pork skins
1 (12 oz.) pkg. roast beef (sub 1-6 oz. pkg. beef brisket)
2 large chip bags

Directions
Remove seeds from peppers and dice them. Combine all ingredients in a large chip bag or double bag and set down in a hot pot to heat for 2 hours. A side of instant potatoes goes nicely with this meal.

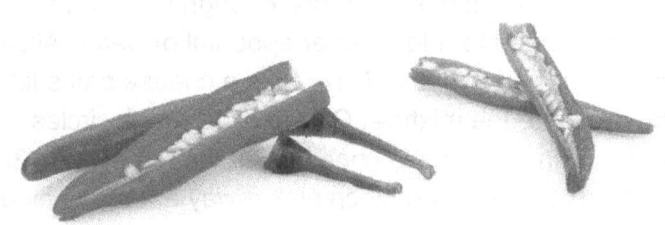

Today, tell yourself:
My stress is decreasing,
and my peace of mind is increasing.

Sweet Treat Chicken

Ingredients
1 (12 oz.) can Sprite
2 (.14 oz.) pkg. lemon-lime electrolytes
1 hot pot insert cup
1 (7 oz.) pkg. chicken chunks
2 hot pots
1 (8 oz.) bag instant white rice
½ coffee mug hot water
1 large chip bag

1 large chip bag
1 large spread bowl
½ (16 oz.) bag tortilla chips

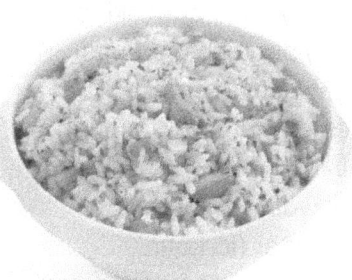

Directions
Combine Sprite and electrolytes in an insert cup. Stir well and set in a hot pot to heat for 45 minutes. In the second hot pot, heat the chicken chunks package for the same amount of time. Once cooking time is up, combine chicken chunks, rice, and hot water in a large chip bag. Add contents from insert cup to the chip bag. Shake well, tie off, and wrap in a towel for 10-12 minutes. Pour into your bowl and use your tortilla chips for dipping.

Today, tell yourself:
It is a joy to relate to myself
and the world around me in
kind and loving ways.

Traditional Tamales

Ingredients
1 (11 oz.) bag party mix
1 (8 oz.) bag jalapeño chips
1 (16 oz.) bag corn chips
1 (16 oz.) bag tortilla chips
2 (2.75 oz.) bags pork skins
1 (11 oz.) bag cheese puffs
4 sleeves saltine crackers
5 pieces cornbread (optional)
2 small trash bags
garlic powder (to taste)
onion powder (to taste)
2 pkgs. chili Ramen seasoning
2 pkgs. spicy vegetable Ramen seasoning
black pepper (to taste)
4-6 large spread bowls
5 coffee mugs hot water
Choice of meat
12 (1.3 oz.) jalapeno peppers
1 (16 oz.) bottle squeeze cheese
32-48 empty Ramen noodle bags

Directions
You may not want to attempt this recipe unless you are an experienced cook. Remove the pretzels from the party mix and set them aside. Crush each bag of chips into a fine powder, including cheese puffs and saltine crackers. Place all in a small trash bag and shake until all is mixed well. If you choose to include cornbread, break it up and add it to the bag as well. Add all your seasonings and shake until all are coated. Divide this mixture into 2-3 large spread bowls. Quickly but carefully add water while kneading. You will want a wet but smooth consistency. You are making masa, and you do not want this to

be too wet. Wet enough that all holds together and spreads without breaking up.

Evenly spread the bowls and equally divide into 16 parts per bowl. Using your ID card works best for this. Each part, when shaped, will be your tamale. Two bowls equal 32, and 3 bowls will be 48 tamales. Set bowls aside for a few minutes before shaping. In a separate bowl, place diced-up choice of meat(s) and jalapeno peppers. Add refried beans to this bowl with 4 cups of hot water, stir, and cover the bowl for 15 minutes. Once cooking time is up, divide this mixture into 2-3 large spread bowls. These will also be divided into 16 equal parts per bowl, so if you have 2 bowls of meat mixture. Three bowls of masa equals 3 bowls of meat mixture.

Now, you can open a trash bag and lay it on your bunk or table. One by one, remove masa from bowls and shape each one into a 4" by 5" shape. Now, remove the meat mixture, one by one, and set it on the masa. Top with cheese and roll up tightly.

Put one tamale into each of your empty Ramen bags. Repeat this process until all your masa and all your meat mixture is gone.

You can eat these just as they are or heat them up using your hot pot. Here is a tip for heating using a hot pot.

Remove and clean your fan cover. Fill your hot pot to the brim. Set the fan cover on top of the hot pot, lip facing up. Put a dozen tamales inside the fan cover, and using a trash bag, cover the fan cover and tie it onto the hot pot. Allow to heat for 2 hours. Now you can see why only an experienced cook should try this recipe. Those do take time but are well worth the time and trouble.

Today, tell yourself:
Yes, I can and
Yes, I will.

Tuna Lasagna

Ingredients
1 (3 oz.) chili Ramen noodle
1 (8 oz.) bag instant white rice
2-1/2 coffee mugs hot water
1 large chip bag
2 (1.3 oz.) jalapeno peppers
1 (9 oz.) pickle
1 (16 oz.) bottle squeeze cheese
black pepper to taste
½ (15 oz.) jar sandwich spread
2 (2 oz.) pkgs. ranch dressing
2 (4.53 oz.) pkgs. tuna
garlic to taste
½ (8 oz.) bag Shabang chips

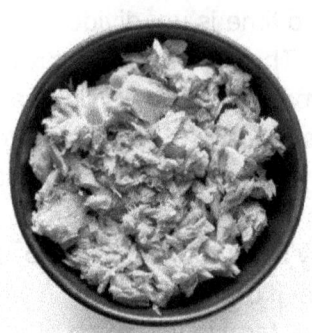

Directions
Combine Ramen, rice, and hot water in a large chip bag. Shake and tie up. Wrap the bag in a towel and set aside for 10-12 minutes. While waiting, dice up peppers and pickles. Once cook time is up, add peppers, pickle, ½ the cheese, pepper, ½ the sandwich spread, 1 ranch dressing, tuna, and garlic to bag and mix well. Very well. Shape in the bag and allow to sit for 10 minutes. Cut the bag open and top it with the remaining cheese and sandwich spread. Now crush chips to top off.

*Today, tell yourself:
I cannot change my past, and I
can't predict the future,
but my gratitude right now can change my present.*

Tuna-Mack-Cocktail

Ingredients
1 (3.5 oz.) pkg. mackerel
1 (4.23 oz.) pkg. tuna
1 large spread bowl
½ (12 oz.) V-8 juice
1/3 (20 oz.) bottle ketchup
1 (1.3 oz.) jalapeno pepper
½ (9 oz.) pickle
1 Tbsp. onion powder
1 tsp. garlic powder
1 pkg. Chili Ramen seasoning
2 Tbsp. hot sauce
1 rice bag
1 sleeve Saltine crackers

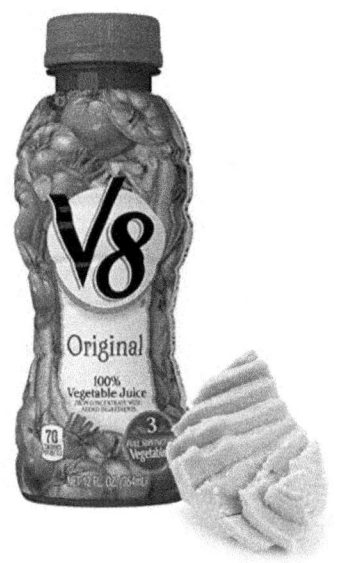

Directions
Combine mackerel and tuna in a large spread bowl. Add V-8 and ketchup to this and stir well. Dice up a jalapeno pepper and pickle. Add these to the bowl along with all seasonings and hot sauce. Mix well and pour the mixture into a rice bag. Set down in a hot pot to heat for 1 hour. Eat with crackers and your favorite drink.

Today, tell yourself:
I will love life and allow life
to love me.

Typical Bean Burritos

Ingredients
1/3 (15 oz.) bag refried beans
1 Tbsp. onion powder
1 tsp. garlic powder
1 pkg. Chili Ramen seasoning
2 coffee mugs hot water
1 large spread bowl
1 (10 oz.) pkg. flour tortillas
2 rice bags
2 hot pots

Directions
Combine refried beans, all seasonings, and hot water in a large spread bowl, mix well, cover, and let sit for 15 minutes. Lay out flour tortillas and coat each one with bean mixture. Roll up and place 4 in each rice bag. Set bags inside hot pots and allow them to heat for 2 hours. You will need to do a second round in one hot pot.

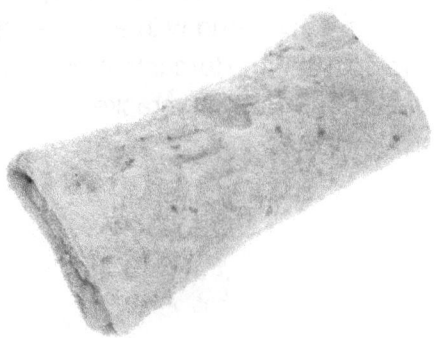

*Today, tell yourself:
I will not worry about what could
go wrong, I choose to focus on
What's going right?*

Wacky-Delish-Sandwich

Ingredients
½ (2 oz.) pkg. vanilla chike (protein powder)
3 Tbsp. instant chili beans
½ (.14 oz.) pkg. orange electrolyte
¼ coffee mug hot water
1 heaping Tbsp. black beans (sub. refried beans)
1 large spread bowl
2 slices wheat bread

Directions
Set bread aside and combine all remaining ingredients in a large spread bowl; stir, cover, and allow to heat for 10 minutes. Spread it on bread and eat it up. I told you it's wacky, and you, too, will say it's delish.

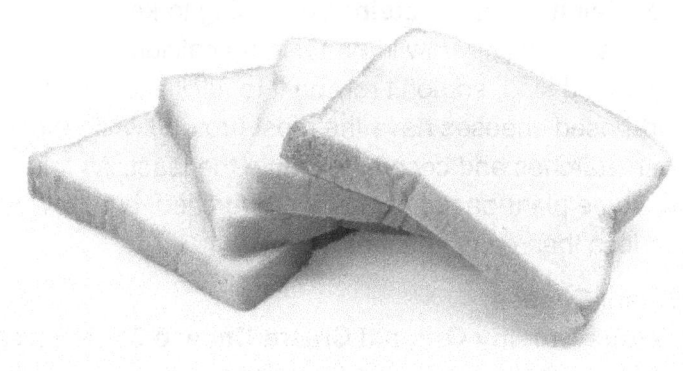

Today, tell yourself:
Each day may not be perfect,
but today will be.

(Vegan) Cheese, Please!

From meltable shreds and sandwich slices to cream cheese, here's what to look for when shopping for a plant-based version and some of the faves.
By Maxine Yeung, M.S. RD, NBC-HW

Screen for Saturated Fat: While dairy-based cheese typically has at least 3 grams of saturated fat per serving, vegan cheese is often made with coconut oil and can have as little as half 7 amount. Look for 6 grams or less per serving- ones made from nuts and seeds that will primarily contain heart-healthy unsaturated fats to help keep your saturated fat intake from exceeding 10% of your total daily calories.

Watch for Sodium: Cheese is inherently salty. Hard varieties, like parmesan, are on the higher side, while cream cheese is on the lower. Aim for 260 milligrams or less of sodium per serving to help stay under 2,300 milligrams a day.

Consider Calcium and Protein: Something to keep in mind: vegan cheese is usually low in protein and calcium compared to the dairy-based kind, so don't rely on it to fulfill those goals. Nut- and seed-based cheeses have the most protein, while those made with starches and coconut oil have the least. As for calcium, some plant-based cheeses are fortified, but they often still have less than dairy versions.

Best Cream Cheese:
So Delicious Creamy Original Cream Cheese Style Spread
70 Cal, 6g sat fat, 0g protein, 115 mg sodium, 0mg calcium
coconut oil makes this super-creamy spread look and feel just like the real thing (minus a little of the tang).

Best Mozzarella:
Vegan Mozza-Shred
80 Cal, 5g fat, 190mg sodium, 0g protein, 0g calcium

Don't be fooled by the drier-looking melt of this mozz-it's plenty gooey. Cheese pull, anyone?

Best Soft Cheese:
Treeline French Style Cheese Herb Garlic
90 Cal, 1g sat fat, 0g protein, 170mg sodium, 140mg calcium
A salty Cheddar is reminiscent of mild dairy versions; it's the best melter of all the ones, perfect for a grilled cheese on top of a plant-based burger.

Best Pepper Jack:
Field Roast Spicy Original Vegan Chao Slices
60 Cal, 4g sat fat, 0g protein, 180mg sodium, 0mg calcium
Dotted with spicy pepper flakes, these creamy slices are good, both cold and melted.

NUMBERS TO LOOK FOR

Saturated Fat
6g

Sodium
260mg

Troy Traylor

History of Pizza

Pizza was first invented in Naples, Italy, as a fast, affordable, tasty meal for working-class Neapolitans on the go. While we all know and love these slices of today, pizza didn't gain mass appeal until the 1940s, when immigrating Italians brought their classic slices to the United States.

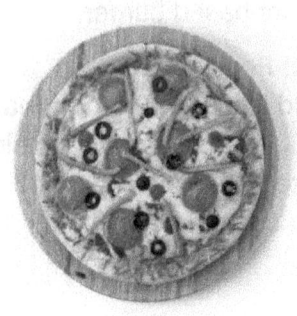

If you think of pizza being quintessentially Italian, you're correct to do so. Italians have been topping flatbread with things for a very long time. There is archeological evidence dating all the way back to 5000 BC indicating that ancient peoples on the Island of Sardinia baked something that could be considered the primordial ancestor of modern pizza. Throughout the region, people ate similar flatbread pizzas, and there is even a reference to flatbread topped with vegetables in the Aeneid.

As far as the word itself is concerned, the first recorded use of the word "pizza" dates all the way back to the 10th century. However, that pizza would really begin migrating out of Italy and across the world.

But what are some of the weirdest things people enjoy on their pizza? There's a restaurant in Michigan that puts zucchini on pizza. As for the rest of the world, here are some common toppings:

In Australia, they like a little shrimp on their pizza. They also enjoy breakfast pizza with eggs, bacon, and other standard morning meal essentials.

Brazil adds some things that will undoubtedly seem strange to pizza purists, including green peas, raisins, and corn.

In Germany, you can add tuna to a pizza. Think open-faced tuna melt!

Much like the standard Greek pizza toppings in the U.S., in Greece, they enjoy olives, feta, and oregano on their pizza.

Indian food is popular in restaurants all over the U.S. If you make your way to India, you can order pizza with some popular local toppings like minced mutton and pickled ginger.

If you're OK with eating eel and squid, Japan has the pizza toppings you're longing for.

Russians like their pizza fishy. Some typical toppings to expect include mackerel, red herring, salmon, and tuna.

In Sweden, pizzas bring warmth to your soul with the addition of curry powder. Bananas and peanuts are also standard options, though the most popular variety is topped with kebab meat.

Whether you stack it up with meats, veggies, seafood, or even more exotic toppings, it's tough to beat a good pizza with a crisp crust and plenty of flavor! So, how do you take your pizza?

Food Facts

Protein

Protein encompasses a large category of complex molecules. It is a macronutrient alongside the other two big ones: carbohydrates and fat. Protein consists of building blocks called amino acids, of which there are around 20 different types that all link up in different combinations. Your body breaks down the various proteins into those amino acids and then recombines them into new proteins to build up your body's muscles. Although your body can make its own amino acids, it can't create all the ones that it needs. The 11 acids your body makes itself are known as non-essential amino acids; the nine that it cannot make are known as essential amino acids. Dietary proteins are found in the following:

> Lean meats- beef, lamb, pork
> Poultry: chicken, turkey
> Fish and seafood: fish, shrimp, crab, lobster
> Eggs
> Dairy products -milk, yogurt, cheese
> Nuts and seeds: almonds, pine nuts, walnuts, hazelnuts, cashews, pecans, pumpkin seeds, sesame seeds, sunflower seeds
> Legumes and beans: beans, lentils, chickpeas, green peas, peanuts, split peas, tofu

How much protein should one eat?

Calculate your daily amount in grams: the standard recommendation is around 7 grams of protein for every 20 pounds of body weight; another is to divide your body weight in half and consume that number in grams of protein. Be aware that your body is only capable of processing so much before it becomes overly saturated and expels any excess protein that it cannot use in your urine. This can be dangerously taxing on your kidneys as you are forcing them to filter out excess protein; several dysfunctional kidney diseases are the result of a high-protein diet, such as kidney stones, just to name one.

When should you eat protein?

This is a hotly contested topic in the health and fitness world, and it's even more vigorously disputed among bodybuilders. One school of thought is that you should eat protein almost immediately post-workout when your body is primed for protein and carbohydrate intake. Yet many dietitians correctly posit that your body is in an ideal state for receiving protein up to three hours after a workout.

Muscle growth

Muscle growth is generated by the stimulation of muscle tissue through exercise. Several studies have shown that bodybuilders and weight trainers will gain muscle mass at the same rate, whether they supplement their diet with extra protein shakes. Remember, your body cannot process more than a certain amount of protein a day, so you won't get "swole" from just drinking chikes. You will, however, get that sculpted look by working out and staying dedicated.

Maintaining muscle mass

As we age past 50 years old, our bodies begin to gradually shed skeletal muscle, a condition known as sarcopenia. Thus, it is even more important for older people to eat protein effectively by consuming high-quality protein foods, such as lean meats or legumes.

Consensus

There is a great deal of misinformation and controversy swirling around protein, but the general recommendation is the common-sense one: don't eat too much, and don't eat too little.

Key Protein Vocabulary

Amino acids are often referred to as the building blocks of proteins and are compounds that play many critical roles in your body. They are needed for vital processes such as building proteins, hormones, and neurotransmitters, and are concentrated in protein-rich foods such as meat, fish, and soybeans.

Carbohydrates (or carbs) are sugar molecules. Along with proteins and fats, carbohydrates are one of the three main nutrients found in foods and drinks. Your body breaks down carbohydrates into glucose. Glucose, or blood sugar, is the main source of energy for your body's cells, tissues, and organs.

Macronutrients are carbohydrates, fat, and protein. They are the nutrients you use in the largest amounts. They are the nutritive components of food that the body needs for energy and to maintain its structure and systems.

Protein is an important part of a healthy diet. It is made up of chemical "building blocks" called amino acids. Your body uses amino acids to build and repair muscles and bones and to make hormones and enzymes. They can also be used as an energy source.

Sarcopenia is a syndrome characterized by progressive and generalized loss of skeletal muscle mass and strength. It is correlated with physical disability, poor quality of life, and death.

Electrolytes

The commissary nearest you offers three flavors of electrolytes. They are fruit punch, lemon-lime, and orange. Within these delicious flavors are calcium, potassium, and magnesium, which our body needs for replenishment. Electrolytes nourish cells, regulate PH levels, and support the nervous, muscular, cardiovascular, and central nervous systems to function properly. They are often talked about in association with dehydration and mentioned in ads for sports drinks that promise to replace electrolytes lost through sweat. So, I urge you to take inventory of how you live and begin to focus on a healthier you! In closing, make sure you stay hydrated this summer.

*Believe in yourself and your potential
If you do, one day, you will tell
your story of how you overcame
and that, my friend, will become
someone else's survival guide.*

Section 7:
Sweets and Treats

Baltimore's Bonbons

Ingredients
1 (16 oz.) pkg. Duplex cream cookies
2 large spread bowls
Approx. 6 Tbsp. water
½ (4 oz.) bag instant milk
½ (12 oz.) bag creamer
3 Tbsp. peanut butter
2 regular-size Snickers bars

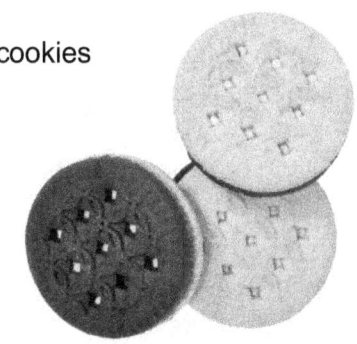

Directions
Separate the cream from the cookies and set the cream aside, as well as 12 vanilla cookie halves. Crush the remaining cookies and place them in bowl #1. Add approximately 3 Tbsp. water to this and knead into a pliable dough. Do not want it too wet, just moist enough so it all sticks together. Flatten the dough out into the bottom of the spread bowl and even it out. Equally, divide this into 12 parts.
In bowl #2, combine milk, creamer, peanut butter, half the cookie cream, and 2-1/2 Tbsp. water and whip until all are incorporated. It will be super thick, but get out all the lumps and clumps.
Flatten out and divide into 12 equal parts. Cut Snickers bars into 6 pieces each.
Set out the 12 vanilla cookie halves. One by one, remove the milk mixture from the bowl, roll each piece into a ball, and put it on top of a half cookie. Lightly push down. Top each one with a piece of a Snickers bar.
Remove dough, one piece at a time, roll each into a ball, and flatten out like a pancake. Drape each one over the cookie halves and pinch around the bottom. Take the remaining cream from the cookies, add a few drops of hot water, and whip. Drizzle a little over each bonbon. Allow you to sit for 1 hour before you eat. That's how we do it in Baltimore.

Troy Traylor

Chocolate Brownies

Ingredients
1 (16 oz.) pkg. Duplex cream cookies
8 chocolate chip cookies
1 large spread bowl
1 (10 oz.) bag hot chocolate mix
5 Tbsp. hot water
1 large chip bag
1 (2 oz.) pkg. cream cheese
1 regular-size Snickers bar
1 regular-size M&Ms

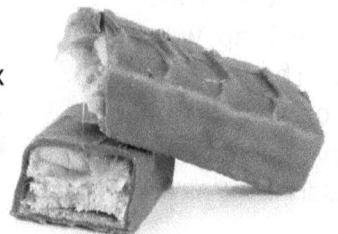

Directions
Separate the cream from the cookies and place the cream aside. Crush Duplex and chocolate chip cookies into a fine powder and place them all in a bowl. Add the hot chocolate mix and water to this and knead into a pliable dough. This will be very thick. Just want it moist enough, so it all sticks together. Once kneaded, place the mixture in the chip bag and flatten it out like you would a pizza. Make it as even as possible and to your desired thickness. Cut the bag open and allow it to dry for 1 hour. While waiting, combine the cream from the cookies, cream cheese, and the Snickers bar together in a hot pot insert cup, and set it down in a hot pot to melt while the brownie dries. Stir occasionally. Once dry time is up, whip the mixture in a hot pot and pour over the brownie. Keep a little from the edge all the way around. Now decorate with a package of M&Ms. Allow this to sit for 45 minutes, cut into ID-size pieces, and serve.

> *Today, tell yourself:*
> *I am a product of my choices, not of my*
> *circumstances and good choices,*
> *they are easy for me to make.*

Chocolate Éclair Soup

Ingredients
1 (3 oz.) Ramen noodles (any flavor)
6 Tbsp. hot chocolate mix
1 coffee mug hot water
1 empty peanut butter jar
15 vanilla wafers

Directions
Crush Ramen and set aside the seasoning package. Combine Ramen, hot chocolate mix, and hot water in a peanut butter jar and shake well. Allow to sit for 5 minutes. While waiting, break wafers into large pieces. After cooking time is up, add wafers to the jar, shake again, and let sit for about 3 minutes before eating. Sounds crazy, I know, but you'll be crazy about the taste once you try it. Save the seasoning package for a spread.

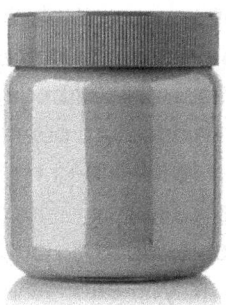

Today, tell yourself:
Good doesn't cut it, I will
strive to be remarkable.

Troy Traylor

Cookie Bars Delight

Ingredients
1 (16 oz.) pkg. Duplex cream cookies
1 hot pot insert
1 (5.6 oz.) pkg. Maria cookies
1 large spread bowl
6 Tbsp. hot water
2 regular-size pkgs. M&M's
1 heaping Tbsp. peanut butter

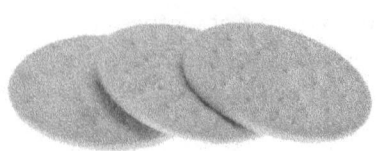

Directions
Separate the cream from the cookies and place the cream in an insert cup. Set the cream aside. Combine Duplex cookies and Maria cookies in a large spread bowl, and use a cup or jar to crush into a fine powder. Add 4-1/2 Tablespoons water to this bowl and knead into a pliable dough. Don't want to be too wet. Crush 1 package of M&Ms and add to the dough, and fold in. Split this mixture into 3 equal parts, and using your cookie tray, press all into slots to form your bars. Even all out. Grab a couple of pieces of white paper or even an old chip bag. Turn the tray upside down and begin pressing in at the end, and work your fingers toward the middle. Bars will begin to fall out. Allow these to sit for 1 hour. While waiting, add peanut butter and 1 Tablespoon of hot water to the insert cup, stir well, and set in a hot pot for 1 hour. Stir occasionally. Once dry time is up, whip the contents into the insert cup and pour over the bars. Allow this to sit for 1 hour before you eat.

Today, tell yourself:
My struggles will end
when my gratitude begins.

Cookie and Cream Bars

Ingredients
1 (16 oz.) pkg. Duplex cream cookies
2 large spread bowls
1 (4 oz.) pkg instant milk
½ coffee mug hot water
2 regular-size Snickers bars

Directions
Separate the cream from the cookies and set the cream aside. Crush cookies into a fine powder and place in bowl #1. In bowl #2, combine instant milk, cream from cookies, and hot water. Whip until all is incorporated, with no lumps and clumps. Once whipped, add cookie powder to the milk mixture and stir/fold until all is mixed thoroughly. Cut up the Snickers bars into small pieces and add to the mix. Now fold again until incorporated. Using the cookie tray, divide your mixture into three equal parts and fill the tray; even out these bars. Lay out some plain white paper and turn the tray upside down. Push bars out and onto the paper, starting at one end and working towards the other end. Allow these bars to set up 2-3 hours before you eat.

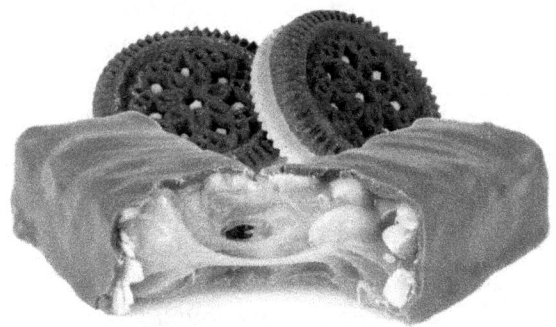

Today, tell yourself:
I will do all that is humanly possible
to sharpen my faith tools.

Troy Traylor

Cranberry Crumble Pie

Ingredients
2 (16 oz.) pkgs. Duplex cream cookies
2 large bowls
12 Tbsps. water
½ (12 oz.) bag creamer
½ (4 oz.) bag instant milk
½ (10 oz.) bag mega omega trail mix
2 individual granola bars

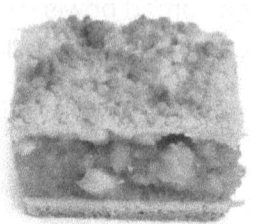

Directions
Separate the cream from the cookies and put the cream in bowl #1. Crush all cookies into a fine powder and place in bowl #2. Add 8 Tablespoons of water to bowl #2 and knead into a pliable dough. Do not want to get too wet. Moist enough so it all sticks together. Flatten out the bottom of the bowl and work it into your pie crust. Set this aside for 1 hour. About 10 minutes before cooking time is up, add creamer and milk to bowl #1 with 5 Tablespoons water and whip until smooth and creamy. Remove cranberry pieces from Mega Omega and hydrate in a little hot water for 5 minutes. Add these to the milk mixture and stir well. Pour this into the pie crust and smooth it out. Crush granola bars and cover the top of the pie. Use a spoon to press into the batter a bit. Allow it to sit for 3-4 hours before you cut and serve.

Today, tell yourself:
I will put the needs of
others before my own.

Excellent Empanadas

Ingredients
2 large spread bowls
4 (5.6 oz.) pkgs. Maria cookies
3/4 (12 oz.) can orange mango juice
4 individual pkgs. sweetener
¼ (12 oz.) bag creamer
¼ (4 oz.) bag instant milk
1 (1 oz.) chick-o-stick
1 (2 oz.) pkg. cream cheese
1 small trash bag or large chip bag

Directions

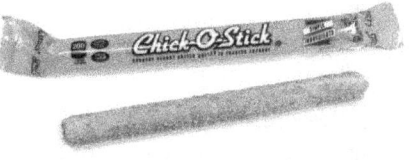

In a large spread bowl, put all the Maria cookies, and using a coffee mug, crush them down to a powder. Some chunks are okay. Pour in a ¼ can of orange mango juice and add two sweeteners. Knead well and roll the mixture into 20 equally sized balls. Set these aside. In a bowl, #2 combine creamer, instant milk, crushed chick-o-stick, two sweeteners, cream cheese, and ¼ can of orange mango juice. Whip well to create a paste-type substance. Take one of your dough balls and flatten it out like a tortilla-like circle. Fill in the middle with a spoonful of mango mix and fold in half (it will look like a half-moon). Crinkle the edges to seal. Can fry on a homemade grill or place in a rice bag and heat in a hot pot for 1 hour. Repeat this process until all ingredients are used up. Enjoy these with hot chocolate or coffee. Your trash bag is used to roll the mixture on.

Today, tell yourself:
I am overflowing with gratitude
and my heart is filled with joy.

Felon Fruitcake

Ingredients

1 (16 oz.) pkg. vanilla cream cookies
2 large spread bowls
1 (.43 oz.) pkg. maple brown sugar instant oatmeal
1 (.43 oz.) pkg apple cinnamon instant oatmeal
1 (2 oz.) pkg. vanilla chike (protein powder)
1 (12 oz.) bag creamer
¾ coffee mug hot water
4 (2 oz.) pkgs. energizer mix
1 small handful of raisins
1 (2 oz.) pkg. cream cheese

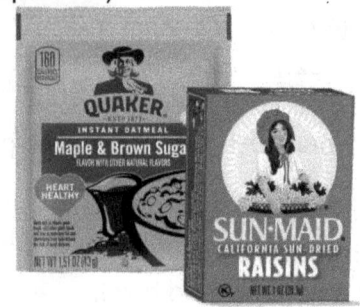

Directions

Remove the cream from the cookies and set the cream aside. Crush all cookies and place them in a large spread bowl. Add both packages of oatmeal to the bowl and lightly stir to mix in. In a separate spread bowl, combine Chike, creamer, and water. Whip this into a thick, creamy substance. No lumps or clumps. Pour this mixture into the cookie mixture and work it until all is incorporated. This should be a thick and sticky substance. Add just three packages of Energizer mix to this and fold until all is mixed in. Flatten out the bottom of this spread bowl and even it out. Cover and let stand for one hour. While waiting, cut up the raisins into smaller pieces and set aside. Using an insert cup, combine the cream from the cookies and the package of cream cheese. Set the insert cup down in a hot pot, unstirred, for your wait time. Once the cake is ready, whip the instant cup, pour it over the top of the cake, and decorate it with raisins and the last package of the energy mix. It's not quite like Grandma makes, but it's pretty good. Let it sit for one hour before you cut and serve.

Holiday Cheesecake

Ingredients
1 (16 oz.) pkg. vanilla cream cookies
2 large spread bowls
1 sleeve golden round crackers (snack crackers)
1 (.43 gram) pkg. maple brown sugar oatmeal
9 Tbsp. water
1 (4 oz.) bag instant milk
1 (2 oz.) pkg. cream cheese
3 Tbsp. creamer
3 holiday pecan pies

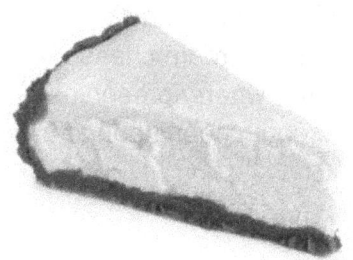

Directions
Separate cream from cookies and put cream in bowl #1. Crush all cookies and crackers and place in bowl #2. Add oatmeal and 5-1/2 Tablespoons water to bowl #2 and knead into a pliable dough. Don't want to be too wet. Moist enough so it all sticks together. May use another ½ Tablespoon water. Once kneaded, flatten out into the bottom of the bowl and work into a pie crust. Set this bowl aside for 1 hour. About 10 minutes before dry time is up, add instant milk, cream cheese, creamer, and 4 Tablespoons water to bowl #1. Whip until all is smooth and creamy. No lumps. Takes a little work. Pour batter into pie crust and level out. Crush holiday pies and cover the top. Allow it to sit for 2 hours before you cut and serve.

Today, tell yourself:
I am grateful for the following 5 reasons...

Troy Traylor

Kiwi-Strawberry-Delight

Ingredients
1 (16 oz.) pkg. vanilla cream cookies
2 large spread bowls
1 (12 oz.) can Kiwi-strawberry juice
1 (.43 grams) pkg. strawberry cream oatmeal
1 (4 oz.) bag instant milk
1 (2 oz.) pkg. cream cheese
4 Tbsp. strawberry preserves
1 pkg. cream cheese pound cakes (2 per package)

Directions
Separate cream from cookies and put cream in bowl #1. Crush all cookies into a fine powder and put in bowl #2. Spoon in 4-1/2 Tablespoons kiwi-strawberry juice into bowl #2 and knead into a dough substance. Now add oatmeal 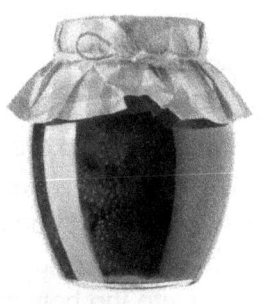 to this mixture and knead again. Flatten the dough out into the bottom of the bowl and even out. Leave it as is, do not make it into a pie crust. Set bowl aside for one hour. About 10 minutes before dry time is up, add instant milk, cream cheese, strawberry preserves, and 4 Tablespoons kiwi-strawberry juice to bowl #1, and, using two spoons, whip until all smooth and creamy. Takes a little work. Pour this into bowl #1 and even out. Crush cream cheese pound cake and sprinkle on top. Use a spoon and press into the batter a bit. Allow this to sit for 4-6 hours before you cut and serve. To beef it up a bit, when serving, add a dollop of strawberry preserve to each piece.

Today, tell yourself:
I will trade my expectations
for appreciations.

No Bake Chocolate Raisin Nut Cookies

Ingredients
1 (10 oz.) bag hot chocolate mix
2 (2 oz.) pkgs. salted peanuts
1 (10 pkg.) box instant oatmeal
2 large spread bowls
1/3 jar peanut butter
18 Tbsp. water
2 good handfuls of raisins
1 small trash bag

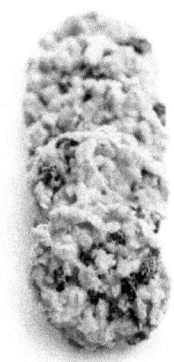

Directions
Set the water aside for a moment. Using both spread bowls, equally, divide all ingredients. Now, one bowl at a time, add 9 Tbsp. water and carefully knead all thoroughly. Once both bowls are kneaded, cover and set aside for an hour to set up and let flavors marry; now flatten the mixture out evenly in each bowl, and using your ID card, divide each bowl into 16 equal parts. Cut the trash bag open and lay it on your bunk or desk. One by one, remove each part from the bowls and flatten out to make cookies. Allow these to sit for 2 hours and eat up. To be a little more creative, if you have cream from cookies available, whip with a few drops of HOT water and top each cookie. These are simply delicious.

Today, tell yourself:
This life is worth living and
I see so much beauty around me.

Troy Traylor

Oh-So-Good-Pie

Ingredients
1 (16 oz.) bag vanilla wafers
1 (6 oz.) bag sunflower seeds
9 Tbsp. water
3 large spread bowl
1 (16 oz.) pkg. Duplex cream cookies
2 (.43 grams) pkgs. maple brown sugar oatmeal
1 heaping Tbsp. peanut butter
1 heaping Tbsp. cappuccino

Directions
Crush vanilla wafers in their bag. Combine wafers, sunflower seeds, and 3 Tablespoons water in bowl #1. Knead this into a pliable dough. Not too wet. Just moist enough so it all sticks together. May need to add a drop or two of water. Flatten out the bottom of the bowl and work into a pie crust. Set aside 1 hour. While waiting, separate the cream from the cookies and place the cream in bowl #2. Set aside a moment. Now, crush Duplex cookies into a fine powder and put all in bowl #3. Add oatmeal, peanut butter, and cappuccino to bowl #3. Mix up. Now add 6 Tablespoons of water to this and work until all is mixed well. It will be super thick. Flatten out in a bowl. Put the cream from the cookies in an instant cup with 1 teaspoon of water, whip, and set in a hot pot to melt. Once dry time is up, run an ID around bowl #3, turn it upside down, and remove the filling. Set this down inside the pie crust and press firmly. Remove cream from hot pot, whip, and pour over pie. Even out and allow it to sit for 30 minutes before you cut. You will see why this is OH-SO-GOOD!

Today, tell yourself:
I can feel it...Today is
the start of something good.

O M G Reese's Replica

Ingredients
1 small cup or bowl
5 heaping Tbsp. hot chocolate mix
3 Tbsp. hot water
3 Tbsp. peanut butter

Directions
In a small cup or bowl, combine hot chocolate mix and water. It will be very thick but whip well. Stir in peanut butter and whip again. Pour it out onto a chip bag or small bowl and shape it into a square. Let sit for 2 hours before you eat. You'll love this one.

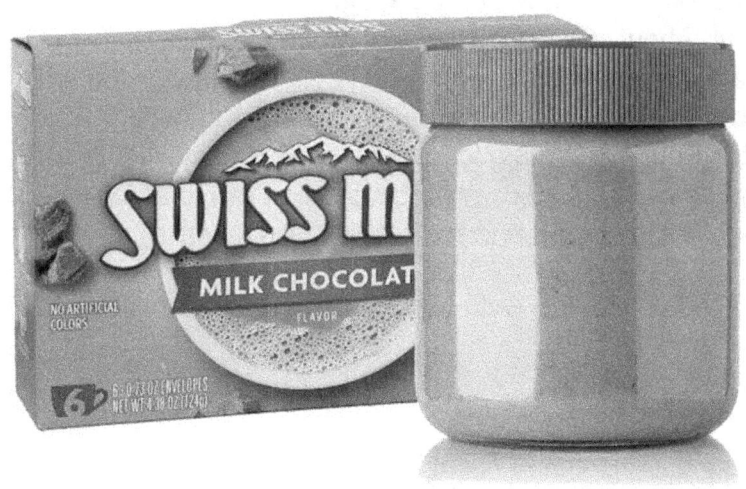

Today, tell yourself:
I love what I see in me.

Troy Traylor

One-of-a-Kind Cheesecake

Ingredients
1 (16 oz.) pkg. strawberry cream cookies
2 large spread bowls
7 Tbsp. Big Red soda
1 (4 oz.) bag instant milk
1 (2 oz.) pkg. cream cheese
1 regular-size M&M peanut

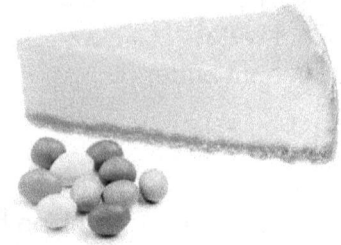

Directions
Separate cream from cookies and place cream in bowl #1. Crush cookies into a fine powder and place them all in bowl #2. Add 4 Tablespoons Big Red to bowl #2 and knead into a pliable dough. Do not want this too wet. Moist enough so it all sticks together. Adjust Big Red as needed. Flatten out the dough into the bottom of the bowl and work it into a pie crust. Set aside for 1 hour. About 10 minutes before drying is up, in bowl #1, add instant milk, cream cheese, and 3 Tablespoons Big Red and whip until all is smooth and creamy. It will be thick, like pancake batter. Pour this mixture into the pie crust and even out. Crush M&M peanuts and decorate the top. Allow this to sit for 4-6 hours before you cut and serve. Will make 8 healthy slices.

*Today, tell yourself:
I welcome the chance to learn,
take risk, make mistakes,
and get up after I fall.*

Fine Dining Prison Cookbook 3

Peanut Butter Cream Delight

Ingredients
1 (16 oz.) Duplex cream cookies
33 Tbsp. peanut butter

Directions
Easiest recipe in the book. Take a package of Duplex cream cookies, open, and top each cookie with peanut butter. What an amazing cookie. To get a little more creative, sprinkle some hot chocolate mix over peanut butter. Either way, this is really good.

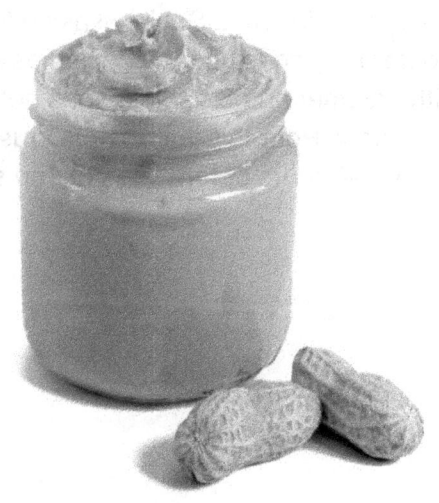

*Today, tell yourself:
In the space between where I
am and where I want to be, I thrive*

Pineapple Cream Pie

Ingredients
1 (16 oz.) vanilla cream cookies
2 large spread bowls
7-1/2 Tbsp. hot water
11 pcs. Pineapple-filled fruit candies
¼ (12 oz.) bag creamer

Directions
Separate the cream from the cookies and put the cream in bowl #1. Crush all cookies into a fine powder and put in bowl #2. Add 4-1/2 Tablespoons hot water to bowl #2 and knead into a pliable dough. Don't want it too wet, just moist enough so it all sticks together. Flatten out the dough into the bottom of the bowl, even out, and work into a pie crust. Set bowl aside for 1 hour. About 10 minutes before drying is up, crush candies and add to bowl #1, along with creamer and 3 Tablespoons hot water. Whip until smooth and creamy. Pour this into the pie crust and even it out. Allow it to sit for 3-4 hours before you cut and serve.

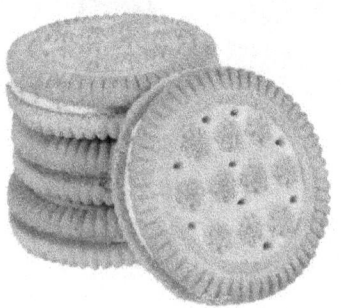

Today, tell yourself:
I have choices and I choose
to do what is right.

Rocky Road Parfait

Ingredients
10 cream cookies (any flavor)
2 large spread bowls
2 Tbsp. peanut butter
1 (10 oz.) bag hot chocolate mix
1 (1 oz.) mint stick
1 regular-size Snickers bar
1 (2 oz.) pkg. salted peanuts
1 regular-size pkg. M&M's
4 individual pkgs. sweetener (sub with 8 tsp. Sugar)
1 empty peanut butter jar

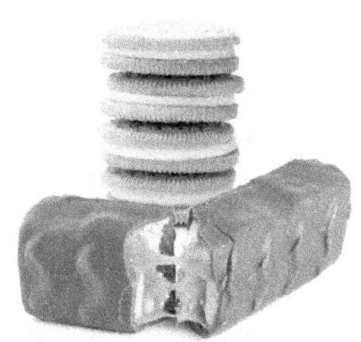

Directions
Separate the cream from the cookies and set the cookies aside. In bowl #1, combine the cream from the cookies and the peanut butter. Whip well. Divide this into 10 equal parts and roll each into a ball. Leave in the bowl and set aside. In bowl #2, combine hot chocolate mix with 3-1/2 Tablespoons hot water and whip for 3 good minutes. Crush the mint sticks and add to the chocolate mixture. Dice up the Snickers bar and lightly crush peanuts. Still leaving peanut butter balls aside, combine all remaining ingredients in bowl #2 and mix well. Now add the peanut butter balls to this and carefully stir in. Pour the mixture, a little at a time, into a peanut butter jar, adding M&M's as you go. Allow this to sit for 2 hours. This is simply delicious.

Today, tell yourself:
I expect all setbacks to turn into comebacks, and all breakdowns to turn into breakthrough this day.

Troy Traylor

Spicy Nut Mix

Ingredients
4 (2 oz.) pkgs. energizer mix
2 (2 oz.) pkgs. salted peanuts
1-1/2 chili Ramen seasonings
1 medium-sized chip bag

Directions
Combine all ingredients in your chip bag and shake well. Once all are coated, it is ready to enjoy. A nice treat for any day.

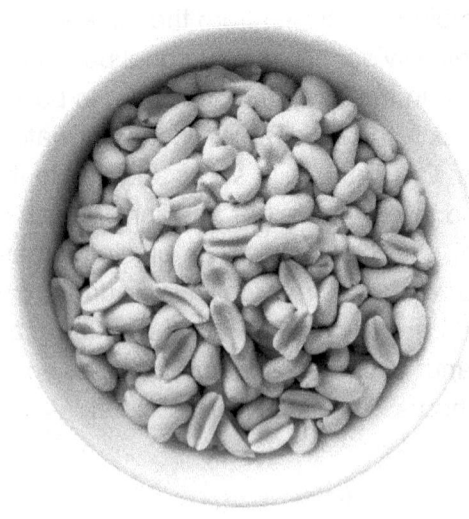

*Today, tell yourself
In all my struggles, I
will find strength and prevail.*

Strawberry-Chocolate Pie

Ingredients
1 (16 oz.) pkg. Duplex cream cookies
2 large spread bowls
1 (.43 grams) pkg. strawberry oatmeal
7 Tbsp. hot water
¼ (10 oz.) bag hot chocolate mix
1 heaping Tbsp. Hazelnut spread
3 Tbsp. strawberry preserves
9 pcs. Strawberry-filled candies

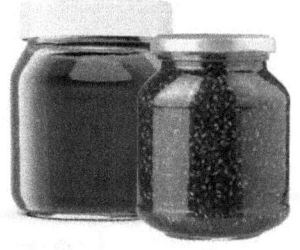

Directions
Separate the cream from the cookies and put the cream in bowl #1. Set aside 6 vanilla cookie halves. Crush the remaining cookies and place them all in bowl #2. Add oatmeal and 4 Tablespoons water to bowl #2 and knead into a pliable dough. Don't want to be wet, just moist enough so it all sticks together. Flatten the dough out into the bottom of the bowl and work it into your pie crust. Set this bowl aside for 1 hour. While waiting, add hot chocolate mix, Hazelnut spread, and strawberry preserves to bowl #2 along with the remaining water. Work on this mixture until all are thoroughly combined. Flatten out in a bowl and allow to sit while the crust dries. This mixture will be super thick. Once drying is complete, remove the mixture from bowl #2. Just use an ID card to loosen the edges and turn them upside down. Set this mixture inside the pie crust and push down firmly. Crush candies and 6 cookie halves. Sprinkle all over the top of the pie and use a spoon to kind of push it into the pie. Allow this to sit for 1 hour before you cut and serve.

Today, tell yourself:
I look backwards with a smile,
and forward with hope.

Troy Traylor

*You don't succeed by being perfect.
You succeed by doing good work,
consistently.*

Section 8:
25 Healthy Choices for the Outside: from the Inside

The recipes in this section have been compiled from family and friends. Some recipes have been first seen in the Taste of Home Magazine, The Echo, The Alvin News, and the Houston Chronicle newspapers.

Baked Feta Spinach-Artichoke Dip

Ingredients
10 oz. frozen cut spinach, thawed and squeezed dry
1 14 oz. can artichoke hearts, rinsed and chopped
2 ½ cups sour cream
1 cup crumbled feta cheese, divided
1 medium shallot, minced
2 cloves garlic, grated
¼ tsp. crushed red pepper
¼ tsp. ground pepper

Directions
1. Preheat oven to 425°F. Coat a 2-quart baking dish with cooking spray.
2. Combine spinach, artichoke hearts, sour cream, ½ cup feta, shallot, garlic, crushed red pepper, and ground pepper in a large bowl. Spread in an even layer in the prepared baking dish. Sprinkle with the remaining ½ cup feta.
3. Bake until lightly browned and bubbly, 25 to 35 minutes. Let cool for 5 minutes before serving. Makes 16: ¼ cup each.

94 Cal, 7g (sat 4g) fat, 24mg Chol, 5g carbs, 2g (added 0g) total sugars, 3g pro, 1g fiber, 147mg sodium, 114mg pot.

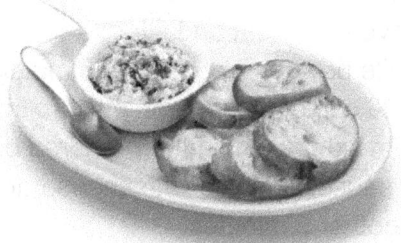

Today, tell yourself:
I will do more smiling and
less worrying, and I will be
more compassionate and less judgmental.

Troy Traylor

Black Bean and Butternut Squash Enchiladas

Ingredients
3 Tbsp. extra-virgin olive oil, divided
3 cups diced peeled butternut squash
2 medium poblano peppers, seeded and chopped
1 medium onion, chopped
1 14oz. can no-salt-added black bean, ringed
4 Tbsp chopped fresh cilantro, divided, plus more for serving
1 tsp. ancho chili powder
8 corn tortillas, warmed
1 10 oz. can enchilada sauce (less than 300mg per serving)
½ cup shredded Monterey Jack cheese
2 cups shredded cabbage
1 Tbsp. lime juice

Directions
1. Preheat oven to 425°F. Lightly coat a 7-by-11-inch baking dish with cooking spray.
2. Heat 2 tablespoons of oil in a large skillet over medium heat. Add squash and cook covered, stirring occasionally, until tender and lightly browned, 8 to 10 minutes. Add peppers and onion and cook, uncovered, stirring occasionally, until tender, about 5 minutes. Remove from heat and stir in beans, 2 tablespoons cilantro, and chile powder. Let cool for 5 minutes.
3. Place about ½ cup of the squash mixture in each tortilla and roll. Place, seam side down, in the prepared baking dish. Top with enchilada sauce. Sprinkle with cheese and cover with foil, and bake for another 5 minutes.
4. Meanwhile, toss cabbage with lime juice, the remaining 1 tablespoon oil, and 2 tablespoons cilantro. Serve the enchiladas topped with slaw and more cilantro, if desired. Serves 4:2 enchiladas and ½ cup slaw each.

428 Cal, 17g (sat 4g) fat, 13mg Chol, 58g carbs, 6g (adding 0g) total sugars, 13g pro, 11g fiber, 491mg sodium, 779mg pot.

> *Today, tell yourself:*
> *This is my day to*
> *live with intention.*

Cashew Chicken Lettuce Wraps

Ingredients

2 Tbsp. canola oil divided
½ cup sliced scallions, plus more for garnish
¼ cup sliced shallot
2 Tbsp. grated fresh ginger
2 lbs ground chicken or turkey
¾ cup unsalted cashews or peanuts, toasted
½ cup thinly sliced celery
½ cup no-salt-added chicken broth
1 Tbsp. cornstarch
2 Tbsp. lime juice, plus lime wedges for serving
2 Tbsp. brown sugar
2 Tbsp. chili-garlic sauce
2 Tbsp. 50%-less-sodium tamari
1 Tbsp. toasted sesame oil
16 leaves Boston or Bibb lettuce
Toasted sesame seeds and thinly sliced bird's eye chiles for garnish

Directions

1. Heat 1 tablespoon canola oil in a large flat-bottom wok or cast-iron skillet over medium heat until shimmering. Add scallions, shallots, and ginger and cook, stirring occasionally, until starting to soften, 2 to 4 minutes. Increase heat to high and add the remaining 1 tablespoon of canola oil and chicken (or turkey). Cook, breaking up with a wooden spoon, until no longer pink and most of the liquids have evaporated, about 8 minutes. Add nuts and celery and cook, stirring occasionally, until the celery is soft, about 3 minutes more.
2. Whisk broth and cornstarch in a medium bowl until smooth. Whisk in lime juice, brown sugar, chile-garlic sauce, tamari, and sesame oil. Add to the pan and cook, frequently stirring, until the sauce thickens, about 3 minutes.

3. Serve about 1/3 cup filling in each lettuce leaf. Garnish with scallions, sesame seeds, and/or chiles, and serve with lime wedges, if desired. Serves 8: 2 lettuce wraps each.

319 Cal, 20 g (sat 4g) fat, 98 mg Chol, 12 g carbs, 6g (added 3g) total sugars, 23g pro, 1g fiber, 281mg sodium, 810mg pot.

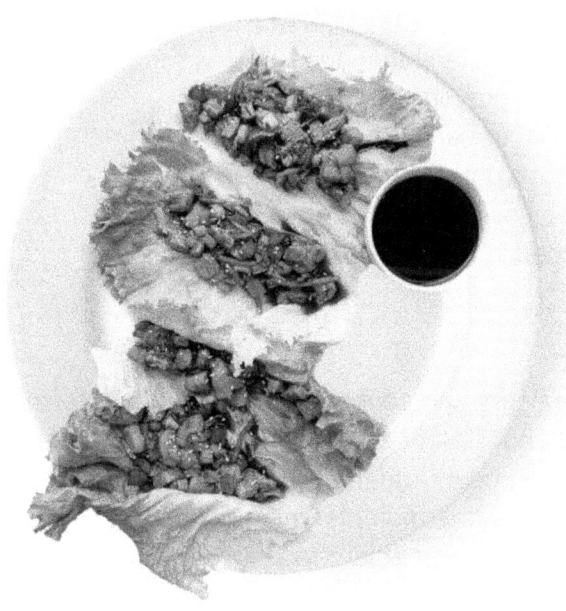

Today, tell yourself:
My joy is my decision,
and today I will be joyful
for and in all things.

Cheesesteak Salad

Ingredients
1 lb. sirloin or cube steak
½ tsp. salt, divided
2 oz. sliced provolone cheese
1 medium red onion, thinly sliced
1 Tbsp. white-wine vinegar
1 ½ tsp. Worcestershire sauce
½ tsp. Dijon mustard
¼ tsp. dried oregano
1 small clove garlic, grated
11 oz. baby spinach
½ cup sliced jarred roasted red peppers, rinsed and patted dry.

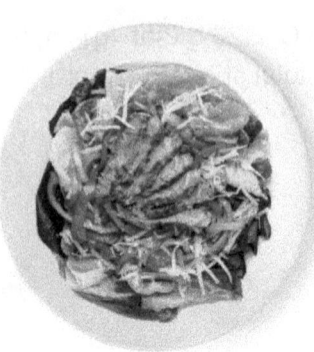

Directions
1. Pat steak dry and season both sides with ¼ teaspoon each salt and pepper. Heat 1 tablespoon of oil in a large skillet over medium-high heat. Add the steak and cook, flipping once, until an instant-read thermometer inserted in the thickest part registers 125°F for medium-rare, 4 to 5 minutes before slicing against the grain.
2. Meanwhile, add onion to the pan and cook, stirring occasionally, until lightly browned, about 5 minutes.
3. Whisk vinegar, Worcestershire, mustard, oregano, garlic, and the remaining ¼ teaspoon each salt and pepper in a large bowl. Slowly whisk in the remaining 2 tablespoons of oil and any steak drippings. Add spinach and peppers and toss to coat. Serve the salad topped with the onions and steak. Serves 4:3 oz. steak, 2 ¼ cups salad and ¼ cup onions each.
342 Cal, 19g (sat 6g) fat, 69mg Chol, 11g carbs, 1g (added 0g) total sugars, 29g pro, 2g fiber, 727mg sodium, 366mg pot.

> *Today, tell yourself:*
> *This life may not always be perfect,*
> *but it sure is beautiful.*

Cheesy Cauliflower and Sweet Potato Chowder

Ingredients
2 Tbsp. extra-virgin olive oil
1 cup chopped onion
½ cup chopped carrot
½ cup chopped celery
2 cups cauliflower florets
1 cup diced sweet potato
2 tsp. chopped fresh thyme
1 bay leaf
½ tsp. salt
½ tsp. ground pepper
¼ cup whole-wheat flour
2 cups low-sodium, no-chicken broth or vegetable broth
2 cups reduced-fat milk
1 cup shredded cheddar cheese, plus more for garnish
¾ cup frozen corn kernels
1 tsp. white-wine vinegar

Directions
1. Heat oil in a large pot over medium heat. Add onion, carrot, and celery; cook, stirring, until soft, about 5 minutes. Add cauliflower, sweet potato, thyme, bay leaf, salt, and pepper. Cook, stirring occasionally, for 3 minutes. Sprinkle flour over the vegetables and cook, stirring for 1 minute. Add broth and milk and bring to a simmer. Adjust heat to maintain a simmer, cover, and cook until the vegetables are soft, about 10 minutes.
2. Stir in cheese, corn, and vinegar. Cook, stirring, until the cheese is completely melted and the corn is hot. It will take about 3 minutes. Discard the bay leaf. Serve sprinkled with more cheese, if desired. Serves 5: generous 1 cup each.

293 Cal, 16g (sat 6g) fat, 30mg Chol, 28g carbs, 10g total sugars (added 0g), 12g pro, 4g fiber, 529mg sod, 584mg pot.

> *Today, tell yourself:*
> *I can't always control what happens on the outside,*
> *but I can always control how I perceive it on the inside.*

Chicken Puttanesca

Ingredients
2 Tbsp. extra-virgin olive oil, divided
4 chicken cutlets (about 1lb.)
¼ tsp. salt, divided
¼ tsp. ground pepper, divided
2 cloves garlic, minced
1 anchovy, minced
¼ cup dry white wine
1 14 oz. can no-salt-added diced tomatoes
¼ cup pitted Kalamata olives, coarsely chopped
1 Tbsp. capers rinsed and coarsely chopped
Chopped fresh parsley for garnish

Directions
1. Heat 1 tablespoon oil in a large skillet over medium-high heat. Pat chicken dry and sprinkle with 1/8 teaspoon each salt and pepper. Add to the pan and cook, flipping once, until browned and an instant-read thermometer inserted in the thickest part registers 165°F, about 6 minutes total. Transfer to a plate.
2. Reduce heat to medium. Add the remaining 1 tablespoon of oil, garlic, and anchovy; cook, stirring, until fragrant, about 30 seconds. Stir in wine, tomatoes, and their juices and the remaining 1/8 teaspoon each salt and pepper. Cook, scraping up and brown bits, until reduced by half, about 10 minutes.
3. Stir in olives, capers, and any accumulated juices from the chicken. Nestle the chicken into the sauce and garnish with parsley. Serves 4:3 oz. chicken and 1/3 cup sauce each.
284 Cal, 13g (sat 2g) fat, 84 mg Chol, 10 g carbs, 6g (added 0g) total sugars, 28g pro, 1g fiber, 466mg sodium, 502mg pot.

> *Today, tell yourself:*
> *Acceptance is the key to*
> *all situations I face.*

Chicken Stew with Collard Greens and Peanuts

Ingredients
3 cups low-sodium chicken broth
2 Tbsp. tomato paste
1 Tbsp. canola oil
½ tsp. kosher salt plus a pinch divided
12 oz. boneless, skinless chicken thighs, trimmed and cut into 1-inch pieces
¼ tsp. ground pepper
1 medium sweet onion, chopped
2 medium carrots, diced
½ medium red bell pepper or 2 mini bell peppers, chopped
3 cloves garlic, finely chopped
1 Tbsp. finely chopped fresh ginger
¼ cup crunchy peanut butter
½ habanero chile or ¼ jalapeno pepper, seeded and finely chopped
1 bay leaf
¼ tsp. ground coriander
1/8 tsp. ground cinnamon
2 cups packed sliced collards or other dark leafy greens
chopped fresh cilantro and unsalted peanuts for serving

Directions
1. Whisk broth and tomato paste in a large measuring cup or bowl until smooth. Set it aside.
2. Heat oil in a large pot over medium-high heat. Season chicken with ½ teaspoon salt and pepper. Add to the pot and cook, turning as needed,

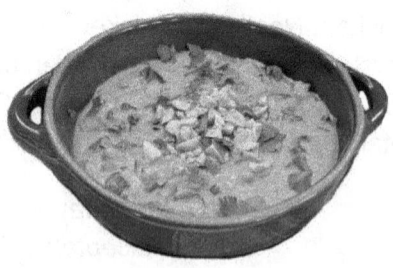

until browned on all sides, about 5 minutes. Transfer to a plate.

3. Add onion, carrots, and bell pepper to the pot; cook, stirring often, until the onion is soft and translucent, 3 to 5 minutes. Add garlic and ginger; cook until fragrant, 45 to 60 seconds. Add the broth mixture, peanut butter, chile pepper, bay leaf, coriander, cinnamon, cumin, and the remaining pinch of salt; stir until smooth. Add the chicken and any juice that has accumulated, squash, and greens.

4. Reduce heat to medium-low, cover, and cook until the vegetables are tender, about 15 minutes. Uncover and cook until the chicken is cooked through and the soup has thickened, about 5 minutes more. Discard the bay leaf. Sprinkle with cilantro and peanuts, if desired. Serves 4: 1-3/4 cups each.
453 Cal, 25g (sat 4g) fat, 80mg Chol, 34 carbs, 12g (added 0g) total sugars, 30g pro, 7g fiber, 608mg sodium, 1.027mg pot.

Today, tell yourself:
I will live this day
as if my life has just begun.

Chili and Garlic Hasselback Squash

Ingredients
1 medium butternut squash (about 2 lbs), peeled, halved lengthwise and seeded
2 Tbsp. water
2 cloves garlic, crushed and peeled
¼ tsp. kosher salt
¼ cup extra-virgin olive oil
1 jalapeno pepper, minced
¼ tsp. ground pepper
fresh cilantro for garnish

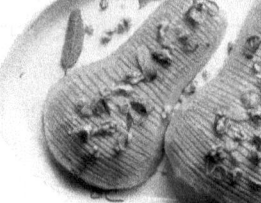

Directions
1. Preheat oven to 425°F. Line a rimmed baking sheet with parchment paper.
2. Place squash in a large microwave-safe bowl and add water. Cover with plastic wrap and microwave on high until just tender, 8 to 10 minutes.
3. Meanwhile, mash garlic and salt together with a fork or a chef's knife on a cutting board, then transfer to a small bowl. Stir in oil, jalapeno, and ground pepper.
4. Lay one squash half, cut side down, between 2 wooden spoons, and make cuts ¼ inch apart, cutting down just to the spoons so the squash stays intact. Carefully transfer to the prepared pan. Repeat with the other half. Brush the oil mixture over the squash, pressing it between each cut.
5. Roast until the squash is lightly browned, 30 to 35 minutes. Serve garnished with cilantro, if desired. Serves 6:1 cup each.
144 Cal, 9g (sat 1g) fat, 0mg Chol, 15mg carbs, 3g (added 0g) total sugars, 1g pro, 3g fiber, 102mg sodium, 458mg pot.

> *Today, tell yourself:*
> *I will take on life today with*
> *an open mind and a grateful heart.*

Cornmeal Crusted Shrimp with Corn and Okra

Ingredients

¼ cup buttermilk
1 Tbsp. hot sauce
½ tsp. garlic powder
2 Tbsp. mayonnaise
1 Tbsp. Cajon seasoning
1 lb. raw shrimp (21-25 count) peeled and deveined
1/3 cup cornmeal
3 Tbsp. extra-virgin olive oil, divided
2 cups frozen corn kernels
2 cups frozen okra
2 cloves garlic, sliced
¼ cup sliced scallions, plus more for garnish
1 Tbsp. butter
1 Tbsp. white-wine vinegar
¼ tsp. salt

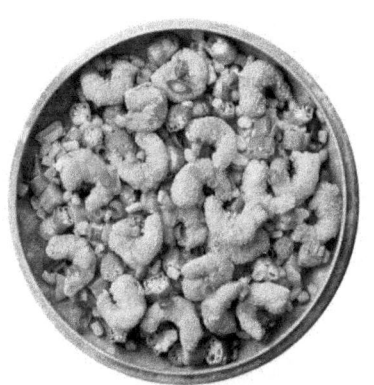

Directions

1. Whisk buttermilk, hot sauce, and garlic powder in a medium bowl. Transfer half the mixture to a small bowl and add mayonnaise. Set aside.
2. Stir Cajon seasoning into the buttermilk mixture in a medium bowl. Pat dry the shrimp and add to the bowl. Toss to coat. Place cornmeal in a shallow dish and dredge the shrimp in it, pressing to adhere.
3. Heat 2 tablespoons of oil in a large nonstick skillet over medium heat. Add the shrimp in a single layer and cook until crispy, about 2 minutes per side. Transfer to a plate.
4. Add the remaining 1 tablespoon of oil to the pan and add the

corn, okra, and garlic. Cook, stirring often, until hot, about 4 minutes. Stir in scallions, butter, vinegar, and salt and toss until well coated, about 1 minute. Serve the shrimp with the vegetables and the reserved sauce. Garnish with more scallions, if desired. Serves 4:3 oz. shrimp, 392 Cal, 20g (sat 4g) fat, 194mg Chol, 28g carbs, 4 g (added 0g) sugars, 27g pro, 4g fiber, 565mg sodium, 532mg pot.

> *The greatest thing in the world*
> *is to know how to belong to oneself.*
> *– Michel de Montaigne*

Fish Tacos Preserved Grapefruit Salsa

Ingredients
1 medium red grapefruit
1 ripe avocado, diced
1 small shallot, minced
2 Tbsp. chopped fresh cilantro
1 Tbsp. preserved grapefruit paste
2 Tbsp. grapeseed or canola oil, divided
1 lb. mild fish fillet, such as cod, halibut, or rockfish
¼ tsp. kosher salt
1 tsp. ground pepper
½ cup shredded cabbage
8 6-inch corn tortillas, warmed

Directions
1. Using a sharp knife, remove the peel and white pith from the grapefruit. Working over a medium bowl, cut. grapefruit segments from their surrounding membranes and any seeds. Add avocado, shallot, cilantro, preserved grapefruit paste, and 1 tablespoon oil; toss to combine.
2. Heat a large cast-iron skillet over high heat. Add the remaining 1 tablespoon of oil and heat until shimmering. Season fish on both sides with salt and pepper. Add to the pan and cook until lightly browned and starting to flake, 2 to 3 minutes per side, depending on thickness.
3. Serve the fish, salsa, and cabbage in tortillas. Serves 4:2 tacos each.
387 Cal, 17g (sat 2 g) fat, 56mg Chol, 35g carbs, 5g (added 0g) total sugars, 25g pro, 7g fiber, 252mg sodium, 861mg pot.

Today, tell yourself:
I will be willing to be
blind to tomorrow, today will
be more than enough.

Ginger Chicken & Vegetable Noodle Soup

Ingredients
2 Tbsp. toasted sesame oil
1 lb. boneless, skinless chicken thighs, trimmed
6 scallions, sliced, whites and greens separated
1-inch knob fresh ginger, peeled
3 cloves garlic, peeled
4 cups low-sodium chicken broth
2 Tbsp. reduced-sodium soy sauce
1 Tbsp. Shaoxing rice wine or dry sherry
1 bunch broccolini, trimmed and halved
6 mini bell peppers, quartered and seeded (2 cups)
2 oz. Chinese egg noodles are broken into small pieces.

Directions
1. Heat oil in an electric pressure cooker in sauté mode. Add chicken and cook, flipping once, until lightly browned, 4 to 6 minutes. Transfer to a plate. Add scallion whites, 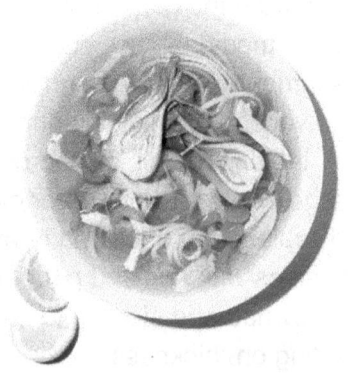 ginger, and garlic to the cooker and cook, stirring until fragrant, about 30 seconds. Turn off the heat.
2. Add broth, soy sauce, Shaoxing (or sherry), and the chicken. Close and lock the lid. Cook on High pressure for 8 minutes.
3. Release the pressure manually. Transfer the chicken to a cutting board and shred it with two forks. Discard the ginger and garlic cloves.
4. Return the cooker to sauté mode and add broccolini, bell

peppers, and noodles. Cook until soft, about 5 minutes. Stir in the chicken. Serves 4:1-1/2 cups each.
337 Cal, 13g (sat 3g) fat, 110mg Chol, 22g carbs, 4g (added 0g) total sugars, 33g pro, 2g fiber, 544mg sodium, 904mg pot.

> *Today, tell yourself:*
> *I will embrace uncertainty and let*
> *life surprise me in many wonderful ways.*

Troy Traylor

Grilled Strawberry Salsa Fresca

Ingredients
1 large, sweet onion
2 jalapeno peppers
2 cloves garlic, unpeeled
1 lb. fresh strawberries, hulled
1/3 cup chopped fresh cilantro
juice of a lime
¼ cup roasted, salted peanuts, coarsely chopped (optional)

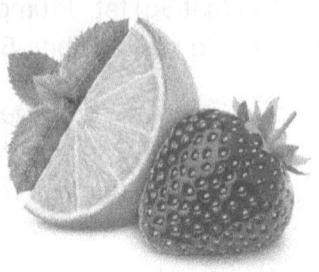

Directions
1. Heat a grill to medium-high. Place a grill pan on the rack. Leaving the root and stem intact, cut the onion into quarters.
2. Grill onion wedges and jalapenos on the grill rack for 5 minutes, turning them brown evenly. Add garlic and strawberries to a hot grill pan. Grill for 5 minutes (10 minutes total for onion and jalapenos), turning frequently, until slightly charred. Transfer strawberries and vegetables to a cutting board; let cool.
3. When cool enough to handle, coarsely chop strawberries and onion. Peel garlic. Finely chop jalapenos (if you like, remove and discard seeds) and garlic. In a bowl, combine berries, onion, jalapenos, garlic, cilantro, lime juice, and ¼ tsp. salt. Cover and chill for 1 hour. If you like, top with chopped peanuts. Serve over grilled chicken or shrimp or with tortilla chips. Makes 3 ½ cups.
per ¼ cup 12 Cal, 43mg sodium, 3g carb, 1g fiber, 1g sugars.

Today, tell yourself:
Gratitude unlocks the fullness of my life.
It turns what I have into enough and more.

Mini Vegan Chocolate Tarts

Ingredients
1 2 oz. pkg. frozen phyllo shells (15 shells)
¼ cup unsweetened coconut milk
6 Tbsp. vegan dark chocolate chips
pinch of kosher salt
mixed fruit for garnish

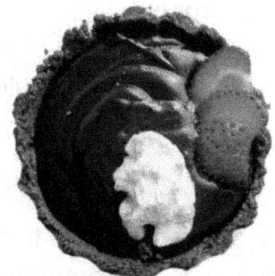

Directions
1. Preheat oven to 350°F.
2. Arrange phyllo cups on a large, rimmed baking sheet. Bake until crisp, 3 to 5 minutes
3. Place chocolate chips and coconut milk in a medium microwave-safe bowl. Microwave on medium for 1 minute 15 seconds. Add salt and stir until smooth. This step is perfect for the kids to do.
4. Fill each phyllo cup with the chocolate mixture and garnish with fruit, if desired. Refrigerate until firm, about 1 hour. This step is also fun for the kids.

Makes: 15 tarts (analysis per tart).
52 Cal, 4g (sat 2g) fat, 0mg Chol, 5g carbs, 2g (added 2g) total sugars, 0g pro, 1 g fiber, 20mg sodium, 52 mg pot.

Today, tell yourself:
I will use all situation I face
to grow my life into a
positive future.

Troy Traylor

Preserved Citrus Paste

Ingredients
1 lb. citrus (about 3 lemons, 5 limes, 2 oranges, or 1 grapefruit), preferably organic
½ cup kosher salt
lemon, lime, or grapefruit juice as needed

Directions
1. Scrub fruit, being sure to remove any stickers. Trim stem ends of lemons, limes, or oranges; trim both ends of grapefruit. Cut the fruit into 1 ½ inch thick wedges.
2. Pack the fruit in a sterilized pint-size glass jar, layering salt between each wedge. Use a wooden spoon to press the fruit down and release the juice, and make room for more fruit. Top off with enough citrus juice to cover the fruit, if needed.
3. Seal the jar tightly with a lid and leave it in a cool place, such as your countertop. Flip upside down once or twice a day for 3 days so that the salt and juice are distributed throughout the jar. You may need to open the jar and press the fruit down to keep it submerged. After a week, transfer the jar to the refrigerator for at least 2 weeks.
4. Rinse the citrus to remove any excess salt. Puree in a blender or food processor. Refrigerate the paste for up to 1 year. Makes about 2 ½ cups (analysis per 1 Tbsp.)
4 Cal, 0g (sat 0 g) fat, 0mg Chol, 1g carbs, 1g (added 0g) total sugars, 0g pro, 0g fiber, 175mg sodium, 20mg pot.

*Today, tell yourself:
In a world where I can be anything
I choose to be grateful.*

Preserved Lemon and Fennel Roast Chicken

Ingredients
1 Tbsp. fennel seeds
1 tsp. crushed red pepper
1 tsp. kosher salt, divided
¼ tsp. ground pepper, divided
2 Tbsp. lemon juice
2 Tbsp. extra-virgin olive oil
2 cloves garlic, minced
1 4–5-pound whole chicken, giblets removed

Directions
1. Combine fennel seeds, crushed red pepper, ½ teaspoon salt, and 1/8 teaspoon pepper in a spice grinder or clean coffee grinder: grind to a powder. Transfer to a bowl and whisk in lemon juice, oil, and garlic until combined.
2. Pat the chicken dry with paper towels. Loosen the skin over the breast and thigh meat and rub the spice mixture under the skin. Sprinkle the remaining ½ teaspoon salt and 1/8 teaspoon pepper on the chicken. Refrigerate, uncovered, for at least 1 hour or up to 8 hours.

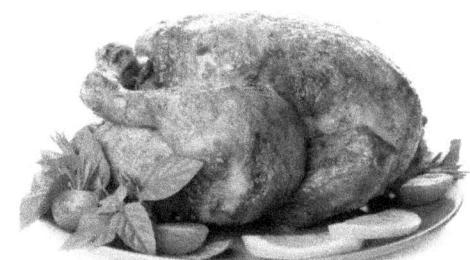

3. Preheat oven to 475°F.
4. Place the chicken breast side up on a wire rack in a roasting pan. Roast for 20 minutes.
5. Reduce oven temperature to 425°F. Continue roasting until an instant-read thermometer inserted in the thickest part of a thigh

without touching the bone registers 165°F, about 40 minutes more.
6. Transfer the chicken to a clean cutting board and let it rest for at least 10 minutes before carving. Serves 8:3 oz. chicken each. 170 Cal, 7g (sat 1g) fat, 78mg Chol, 1g carbs, 0g (added 0g) total sugars, 24g pro, 0g fiber, 374mg sodium, 310mg pot.

> *Today, tell yourself:*
> *Life don't always have to be*
> *a bowl of cherries, but it*
> *also, doesn't have to be a bowl of lemons.*

Red Lentil Soup with Saffron

Ingredients

3 Tbsp. extra-virgin olive oil
2 medium carrots, finely diced
2 stalks celery, finely diced
1 large onion, finely diced
3 cloves garlic, minced
1 Tbsp. tomato paste
½ tsp. ground turmeric
4 cups low-sodium, no-chicken, or chicken broth
1 ½ cups water, plus more as needed
1 lb. red lentils (2 cups), pickled over and rinsed
5 oz. spinach, coarsely chopped
1 tsp. kosher salt
1 tsp. ground pepper
Plain yogurt & chopped fresh mint for garnish

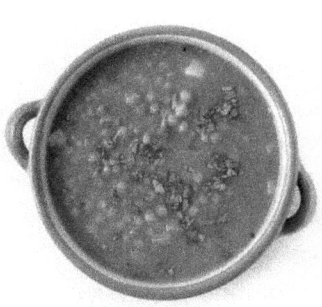

Directions

1. Heat oil in a large, heavy pot over medium heat. Add carrots, celery, and onion and cook until starting to soften, 7 to 10 minutes (do not brown). Stir in garlic, tomato paste, cumin, saffron, and turmeric, and cook for 1 minute.
2. Add broth, water, lentils, salt & pepper. Bring to a simmer, cover, and cook, stirring as needed to prevent sticking, until the lentils and vegetables are tender, 15 to 20 minutes. Add more water if desired.
3. Garnish with yogurt and mint, if desired. Serves 8: generous 1 cup each.
280 Cal, 7g (sat 1 g) fat, 0mg Chol, 42g carbs, 2g (added 0g) total sugars, 15g pro, 8g fiber, 364mg sodium, 512mg pot.

Today, tell yourself:
I have too many flaws to be perfect.
But I have too many blessings to be ungrateful.

Troy Traylor

Roasted Strawberry Frozen Yogurt

Ingredients
1 lb. fresh strawberries, hulled
2 Tbsp. sugar
1 tsp. vanilla bean paste or vanilla
3 cups plain whole milk yogurt
2/3 cup honey
2 Tbsp. light corn syrup
1 cup crushed pretzels and/or crushed freeze-dried strawberries (optional)

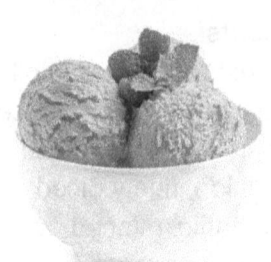

Directions
1. Preheat oven to 300°F. Line a rimmed baking sheet with parchment paper. Place strawberries, sugar, and vanilla bean paste on the baking sheet; gently toss to combine. Roast for 30 to 40 minutes or until berries are very tender and juicy. Let cool to room temperature (45 minutes). Using a potato masher or fork, coarsely mash cooled berries.
2. In a large bowl, stir together plain yogurt, honey, corn syrup, and ¼ tsp. salt. Add the mashed berry mixture to the yogurt; mix well. Cover; refrigerate 4 to 24 hours or until very cold.
3. Freeze the yogurt mixture in a 1 ½ to 2-quart ice cream freezer according to the manufacturer's directions. Transfer to a freezer container and freeze for 2 to 4 hours or until firm.
4. If you like, serve with pretzels and/or freeze-dried berries. Makes 5 cups.
Per ½ cup 157 Cal, 3g fat (2g sat fat), 11mg Chol, 101mg sodium, 32g carb, 1g fiber, 31g sugars, 3g pro.

> *Today, tell yourself:*
> *Love, joy, and sincere gratitude*
> *are a natural part of who I am!*

Roast Salmon with Kumquat-Pineapple Chutney

Ingredients
1 Tbsp. canola oil
½ cup finely diced red onion
10 oz. Kumquats-sliced and seeded
2 cups diced pineapple
½ cup golden raisins
¼ cup white-wine vinegar
1/3 cup lemon juice
4 Tbsp honey, divided
½ tsp. ground coriander
1 Birds Eye Chile, sliced
1 tsp. ground pepper, divided
¾ tsp. salt, divided
2 ½ lbs. skin-on salmon fillet

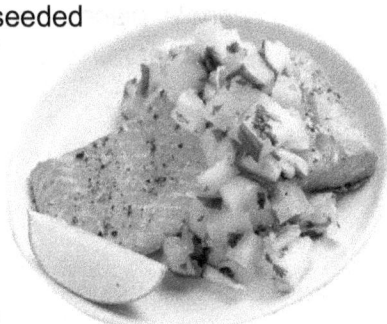

Directions
1. Position the rack in the upper third of the oven; preheat to 450°F.
2. Heat oil in a medium saucepan over medium heat. Add onion and cook, stirring often, until softened, about 5 minutes. Add kumquats, pineapple, raisins, vinegar, lemon juice, 2 tablespoons honey, coriander, chili, and ½ teaspoon each pepper and salt. Bring to a boil. Adjust heat to maintain a simmer and cook, often stirring, until the chutney has thickened, about 15 minutes.
3. Meanwhile, pat the salmon dry and place on a rimmed baking sheet, skin-side down; stir mustard, the remaining 2 tablespoons honey, ½ teaspoon pepper, and ¼ teaspoon salt in a small bowl and brush over the salmon. Bake until the salmon is almost done, 8 to 12 minutes, depending on thickness. Switch the broiler to high and broil until the salmon is lightly browned and flakes easily with a fork, about 3 minutes. Serve with chutney.

Serves 8:4 oz. salmon and 1/3 cup chutney each.
332 Cal, 8g (sat 2g) fat, 78 mg Chol, 30g carbs, 22g total sugar (added 8g), 35g pro, 4g fiber, 352mg sodium, 853mg pot.

> *Today, tell yourself:*
> *I will fill my life with*
> *people, places, and conversations*
> *that make me feel good.*

Saffranskaka (Saffron Cake)

Ingredients
10 Tbsp. (1 ½ sticks) unsalted butter
¼ teaspoon crushed saffron threads
3 large eggs
1 1/2 cups granulated sugar
2/3 cup low-fat milk
6 Tbsp. canola or extra-virgin olive oil
1 cup all-purpose flour
1 cup whole-wheat pastry flour
½ cup almond flour
1 Tbsp. baking powder
pinch of salt
½ cup golden raisins
½ cup sliced almonds, toasted
confectioner's sugar for dusting

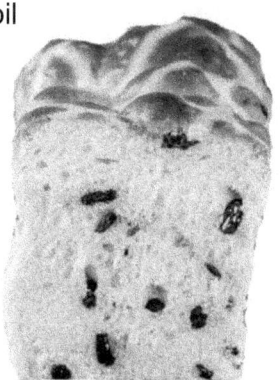

Directions
1. Preheat oven to 350°F. Coat a 9-inch springform pan with cooking spray, line it with parchment paper, and spray again.
2. Melt butter in a medium saucepan over low heat and add saffron. Set aside to cool slightly.
3. Meanwhile, beat eggs and granulated sugar in a large bowl with a hand mixer or stand mixer fitted with the whisk attachment on high speed until pale yellow, about 3 minutes. With the mixer on low, add milk, oil, and saffron butter. Mix for 1 minute. Whisk all-purpose flour, whole wheat flour, almond flour, baking powder, and salt in a medium bowl. Stir into the batter using a flexible spatula. Stir in raisins. Pour the batter into the prepared pan.
4. Bake until a toothpick in the center comes out clean, 45 to 60 minutes. Let cool for 10 minutes. Run a knife around the pan edge and unmold the cake onto a wire rack. Cool completely, about 1 hour. Top with almonds; dust with confectioners' sugar,

if desired. Serves 16:1 slice each.
315 Cal, 17g (sat 6g) fat, 54mg Chol, 37g carbs, 20g (added 16g) total sugars, 5g pro, 3g fiber, 120mg sodium, 150mg pot.

> *Today, tell yourself:*
> *The secret to having it all*
> *is knowing you already do.*

Saffron Chicken Forma

Ingredients
5 Tbsp. canola, avocado, or grapeseed oil divided
5 cups thinly sliced onions
1/4 cup unsalted cashews
¼ cup water
1 ½ cups low-fat plain yogurt
2 tsp. garam masala
½ tsp. ground cardamom
½ tsp. cayenne pepper
½ tsp. ground coriander
½ tsp. ground turmeric
¼ tsp. crushed saffron threads
½ tsp. black peppercorns, crushed
1 bay leaf
1 cinnamon stick
2 lbs. boneless, skinless chicken thighs, trimmed and cut into 2-inch pieces
2 Tbsp. grated fresh ginger
1 cup low-sodium chicken broth
1 tsp. kosher salt
coarsely chopped fresh cilantro for garnish

Directions
1. Heat 4 tablespoons of oil in a large skillet over medium-low heat. Add onions and cook, stirring frequently, until caramelized and slightly crispy, 25 to 30 minutes. Transfer to a blender and add cashews and water. Blend until smooth.
2. Combine yogurt, garam masala, cardamom, cayenne, coriander, turmeric, and saffron in a medium bowl. Set aside.
3. Place the pan over medium heat and add the remaining 1 tablespoon of oil. Add peppercorns, bay leaf, and cinnamon stick and toast until fragrant, 10 to 15 seconds. Add chicken, garlic, and ginger and cook, stirring occasionally, until the chicken starts to brown, 5 to 7 minutes.

4. Stir in the pureed onion mixture, the yogurt mixture, broth, and salt. Adjust heat to maintain a low simmer, partially cover, and cook until the chicken is tender and reaches an internal temperature of 165°F, about 20 minutes. Discard the bay leaf and cinnamon stick. Garnish with cilantro, if desired.

Today, tell yourself:
I will remain grateful for
what I have and, in the end,
I will have more.

Seven-Layer Chicken Burrito

Ingredients
1 cup refried beans
1 ½ tsp. Chipotle chiles in Adobo sauce, finely chopped
4 10-inch flour tortillas
2 cups shredded chicken
¼ cup salsa
½ cup guacamole
½ cup sour cream
1 tomato, chopped
1 cup spinach
½ cup (2 oz.) shredded cheddar cheese
¼ cup black olives, sliced

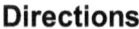

Directions
1. In a small bowl, stir together refried beans and 1 teaspoon of Chipotle chiles. Spread over tortillas. Top each with ½ cup of chicken, 1 tablespoon of salsa, and 2 tablespoons of guacamole. In a small bowl, stir together sour cream and the remaining ½ teaspoon Chipotle chiles. Spoon over guacamole and top with tomato, spinach, and black olives.
2. Roll up burritos and serve with additional salsa if you like. Makes 4.
Per Burrito: 539 Cal, 23g (sat 9g) fat, 90mg Chol, 4g sugars, 34g pro.

Today, tell yourself:
Today will be another great day.

Troy Traylor

Small-Batch Crispy Chocolate Chip Cookies

Ingredients
2 Tbsp. unsalted butter, at room temp.
2 Tbsp. granulated sugar
2 Tbsp. turbinado sugar
1 Tbsp unsweetened applesauce
¼ tsp. vanilla extract
4 Tbsp white whole-wheat flour
¼ tsp. baking soda
1/8 tsp. kosher salt
3 Tbsp. dark chocolate chips

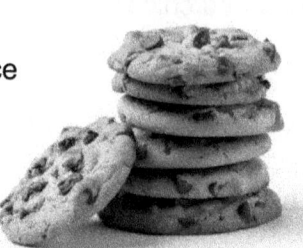

Directions
1. Preheat oven to 350°F. Line the baking sheet with a nonstick silicone baking mat or parchment paper.
2. Combine butter, granulated sugar, and turbinado sugar in a small bowl. Using a rubber spatula, stir until well blended. Add applesauce and vanilla; stir to combine. Add flour, baking soda, and salt; stir to combine. Add chocolate chips and stir to combine. Using a tablespoon measure, scoop the dough onto the prepared baking sheet, spacing cookies about 2 inches apart.
3. Bake until the cookies are golden around the edges, about 8 minutes. Let cool on the pan for 5 minutes, then transfer to a rack to cool and firm up for about 10 minutes.

Makes: 8 cookies (analysis per cookie)
97 Cal, 5g (sat 3g) fat, 8mg Chol, 13g carbs, 9g (added 9g) total sugars, 1g pro, 1g fiber, 70mg sodium, 17mg pot.

Today, tell yourself:
My gratitude and attitude
is not a challenge, it is a choice.

Smoked Trout Potato Salad

Ingredients
1 medium English cucumber, thinly sliced
1 shallot, thinly sliced
¼ cup fresh dill, chopped
¼ cup white wine vinegar
4 cups mixed salad greens
1 pint deli potato salad
2 8 oz. pkgs. smoked trout, skinned, and flaked.

Directions
1. For pickled cucumber: In a small bowl, combine cucumber, shallot, dill, vinegar, and 1 teaspoon salt. Let it stand for 20 minutes.
2. Pile greens and potato salad on 3 plates; top with trout and pickled cucumber.
Serves 4
Per serving: 309 Cal, 14g (sat 3g) fat, 105 mg Chol, 1,524 mg sodium, 20g carbs, 2g sugars, 20g pro.

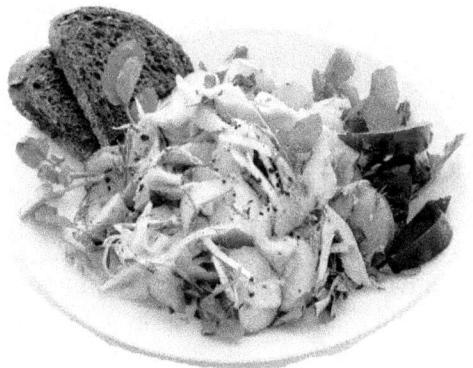

Today, tell yourself:
I am falling in love
with the journey of life.

Southwest Chopped Salad with Tomatillo Dressing

Ingredients
½ cup diced tomatillos
½ cup fresh cilantro leaves
2 small cloves garlic, crushed and peeled
1 Tbsp. finely chopped seeded jalapeno pepper
1/3 cup extra-virgin olive oil
2 Tbsp. distilled white vinegar
1 Tbsp. lime juice
2 Tbsp. agave syrup
¾ tsp. kosher salt
1/4 tsp. ground cumin
4 cups chopped red cabbage
1-1/4 cups thinly sliced, slender multicolored carrots
1 medium yellow bell pepper, diced
1 cup diced peeled jicama
1 cup small grape tomatoes, halved
1 15 oz. can no-salt-added red, black, or pinto beans, rinsed
1 cup diced pepper Jack cheese
1 ripe avocado, diced
lightly crushed corn chips (optional)

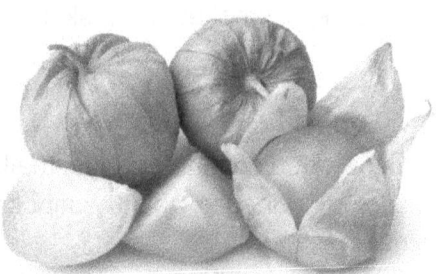

Directions
1. Combine tomatillos, cilantro, garlic, jalapeno, oil, vinegar, lime juice, agave, salt, and cumin together in a blender. Process until smooth.
2. Place cabbage, carrots, bell pepper, jicama, tomatoes, beans, and cheese in a large bowl. Add the dressing and toss to coat. Scatter avocado over the top and garnish with corn chips, if desired. Serves 4: 2 ½ cups each.

519 Cal, 37g (sat 9g) f at, 25 mg Chol, 37g carbs, 11g (added 3 g) total sugars, 15g pro, 14 g fiber, 612 mg sodium, 1051 mg pot.

*Today, tell yourself:
I will be glad and rejoice
in all things, both big and small.*

Tofu Cauliflower & Sweet Potato Green Curry

Ingredients
2 Tbsp. peanut oil
1 14-ounce pkg. extra-firm tofu drained and cut into 1-inch pieces
2 Tbsp. green curry paste (see directions)
1 14-ounce can light coconut milk
1 Tbsp. fish sauce
3 cups cauliflower florets
1 medium sweet potato, cut into 1-inch pieces
2 scallions, sliced, whites and greens divided
1 Tbsp. lime juice, plus lime wedges for serving
Chopped fresh cilantro for garnish

Directions
1. Heat oil in a large flat-bottom wok or cast-iron skillet over medium heat. Pat tofu dry and add to the pan. Cook in a single layer until browned on the bottom, about 4 minutes. Gently stir and continue cooking, stirring occasionally, until browned on both sides, about 4 minutes more. Transfer to a plate.
2. Add curry paste to the pan and cook, stirring for 1 minute. Stir in coconut milk and fish sauce and bring to a simmer. Add cauliflower, sweet potato, and scallion whites. Reduce heat to maintain a simmer, cover, and cook until the vegetables are tender, 12 to 14 minutes. Stir in the tofu and lime juice.
3. Garnish with scallion greens and cilantro and serve with lime wedges, if desired. Serves 4:1 ¾ cups each.

284 Cal, 18g (sat 7 g) fat, 0mg Chol, 18g carbs, 5g total sugars (added 0 g), 14 g pro, 6g fiber, 795 mg sodium, 388 pot.

Today, tell yourself:
Calm, clarity, and peace of mind
are a natural part of my life.

Focus on the Food

Nutrition Facts	
About 8 servings per container	
Serving Size 16 Crackers	(31g)
Amount per serving	
Calories	
	% Daily Value
Total Fat	8%
Saturated Fat	5%
Trans Fat 1g	
Polyunsatured Fat 3g	
Monounsaturated Fat 1g	
Cholesterol 0mg	0%
Sodium 200mg	9%
Total Carbohydrate 23g	8%
Dietary Fiber 3g	11%
Total Sugars 5g	
Includes 5g Added Sugars	10%
Protein 2g	
Vitamin D 0mcg 0% *Calcium 17mg 2%	
Iron 1 mg 8% *Potassium 99mg 2%	
*The % Daily Value (DV) tells you how much a nutrient in a serving of food contributes to a daily diet. 2,000 calories a day is used for general nutrition advice.	
Ingredients: WHOLE GRAIN WHEAT FLOUR, SOYBEAN OIL AND/OR PALM OIL, SUGAR, CORNSTARCH, MALT SYRUP (FROM BARLEY), REFINERS SYRUP, SALT, LEAVENING, (SODIUM BICARBONATE AND AND MONOCALCIUM PHOSPHATE)	

Watch Serving Size

All nutritional labels will reflect value per serving. Be mindful of how many servings are in each package.

Be Heart Healthy
Reducing the amount of sodium in your diet can decrease high blood pressure.

Up Your Fiber
Look for whole-grain options to increase your daily fiber intake. High fiber options can include:
- Wheat Thins
- Oatmeal
- Brown Rice

Sweet Tooth?
Consuming less added sugars can help control diabetes, weight loss, and overall improve dental health.

Look For These Healthier Items at Your Unit Commissary or Local Market

Healthier Foods and Snacks

- Brown Rice
- Instant Oatmeal
- Mackerel Fillets
- Siracha Mackerel
- Tuna in Water
- Tuna with Jalapenos
- Chicken Chili with Beans
- Chicken Chunk in Broth
- Pink Salmon
- Honey Pepper Turkey Bites
- Energizer Mix
- Salted Peanuts
- Granola Bars
- Omega Trail Mix
- Pretzels

Healthier Beverages

- Chocolate Nutrition Shake
- Vanilla Nutrition Shake
- Vanilla Chike Protein Powder
- Strawberry Nutrition Shake
- Orange Juice
- Strawberry/Kiwi
- Pineapple/Orange Juice
- Diet Green Tea with Citrus
- Diet Coke
- Coke Zero
- Lemon/Lime Electrolyte
- Orange Electrolyte
- Fruit Punch Electrolyte

Sugar-Free Options

- Assorted Fruit Candy
- Berry Blue Typhoon Drink Additive
- Wild Purple Smash Drink Additive
- Hot Chocolate

Low Sodium Options

- Chicken Noodle Ramen
- Chili Noodle Ramen
- Spicy Vegetable Ramen
- Chili, No Beans
- Chili with Beans

"Do or do not.
There is no try."
-Yoda,
Jedi Master

Weather Watch

Recognition of cold-related illness, injury

Watch for the following symptoms of frostbite.

- Cold, white, and hard skin;
- Itching;
- Pain;
- Loss of feeling in the affected area;
- Swelling and blistering;
- Skin becomes red and blotchy when warmed; and
- Tissue loss, depending on the severity of the frostbite.

Watch for the following symptoms of hypothermia

- Confusion;
- Drowsiness;
- Slurred speech;
- A drop in blood pressure;
- Shallow breathing; and
- A pinkish tint to the skin.

Tips for prevention and recognition of heat illness

Higher risk conditions for heat illness include:

- A newly assigned job that is highly stressful.
- Receiving psychiatric medications or certain other medications or having certain medical conditions.
- Being elderly.
- High temperatures and humidity
- No significant breeze.

Prevention of heat illness includes:

- Increasing frequency of fluid intake when working in hot environments
- Supplemental water should be available.
- Take a break every 30-60 minutes.
- Decreasing the intensity of work under extreme conditions.
- Access to cold water showers.
- Access to respite areas.
- Allowed fans for all residents.
- Following preventative measures on heat posters.

Types of heat illness:

Heat Cramps: Can be painful and intermittent, involving involuntary muscle spasms following hard physical work or exercise in a hot environment. Cramps usually occur after heavy perspiration and typically occur in the abdomen, arms, and legs. The cause is inadequate replacements of electrolytes (sodium and potassium).

Heat Exhaustion: The most common form of heat illness is caused by the depletion of water and salt. Symptoms include weakness, anxiety, fatigue, dizziness, headache, and nausea. Signs include profuse perspiration and rapid pulse and breathing. Confusion or loss of coordination may also be present. Heat exhaustion, if not treated, may lead to heat stroke.

Heat Stroke: While it may be preceded by signs of heat exhaustion, the onset of heat stroke is often sudden. Symptoms include diminished or absent perspiration and hot, dry, and flushed skin. Other conditions that may be present include increased body temperatures, delirium, convulsions, seizures, rapid pulse, weakness, headache, mental confusion, dizziness, extreme fatigue, nausea/vomiting, and incoherent speech progressing to coma. Medical care is urgently needed. Death may result if left untreated.

Treatment: Seek medical attention as soon as possible. Move the person out of direct sunlight into an air-conditioned environment, if possible, remove clothing while maintaining modesty, and provide water to drink if conscious. Liberally apply cold water on them, and if possible, fan them if there is no breeze.

Access to Respite Areas: During times of extreme temperatures, you must be allowed access to respite areas. Your employer must be trained to be compliant with heat precaution procedures, including knowledge of respite area locations and resident access. The location should be posted at job sites. If you are not at work, you should make yourself aware of cool spots while out in extreme heat.

Closing

This is the third and final book in "Fine Dining Prison Cookbook." My deepest level of gratitude goes out to everyone who has purchased these books and shared their thoughts with me and others.

It has brought me a great amount of joy to know I have been able to produce something that has touched many lives and, of course, stomachs.

I do hope you have found a new level of strength as you continue your journey of life. Times and people are changing, and I feel that our world needs so many more to share positive encouragement and inspire those around them to be the best version of themselves. Some may not even know that version yet, and some may have discovered this version as they read this book.

I would just like to share that my writings have helped me, and I'd like to think that my writings have helped you. Over the years of writing, I have been truly blessed with meeting some amazing people, and I now know what it is like to put others first.

I will remain prayerful that anyone who struggles is able to find strength and those who are filled with strength use it to help others up. With today's society being what it is, I just ask everyone to offer another a hand up and help them find the strength you are filled with.

May you move forward in life with an open mind and open heart. May all your dreams and desires bring you peace, joy, and happiness that last forever. Every day offers a new chance to make this choice. And just so you know, you now have a choice.

Yours truly,

Troy Neal Traylor, Sr.

Your Shopping List

All the ingredients listed are for the first 75 recipes in this book (commissary purchased items). For the "25 Healthy Choices for the Outside, From the Inside," once you choose your recipe(s), just add the ingredients to your next grocery list.

Sizes for commissary items may vary from state to state, so you may need to make some adjustments as needed. If you find any ingredients that are not available to you, don't be afraid to make substitutions.

I am hopeful you can appreciate my time, effort, and, of course, recipes. It has been my pleasure to share all my writings with you. Good luck, stay strong, and remain positive in your daily life.

Candy/Pastries

Candy Bars	Regular Size
Chick-o-Sticks	1 oz. Single
Cream Cheese Pound Cake	2 per Pkg.
Fireballs	10 oz. Bag
Fruit-Filled Hard Candy	8 oz. Bag
Fruit/Mint Sticks	1 oz. Single
Holiday Pecan Pies	2 oz. Pkg.
M & M's	Regular Size

Chips/Crackers

BBQ Chips	8 oz. Bag
Cheese & Chive Crackers	1.375 oz. Pkg.
Cheese Puffs	11 oz. Bag
Corn Chips	16 oz. Bag
Golden Round Crackers	Sleeves
Jalapeno Chips	8 oz. Bag
Nacho Chips	3 oz. Bag

Matzo Crackers	16 oz. Box
Packaged Crackers	1.375 oz. Pkg.
Party Mix	11 oz. Bag
Pork Skins	2.75 oz. Bag
Regular Potato Chips	2 oz. Bag
Saltine Crackers	Sleeves
Shabang Chips	8 oz. Bag
Small Chips	2 oz. Bag
Snack Crackers	Sleeves
Tater Skins	8 oz. Bag
Tortilla Chips	16 oz. Bag

Condiments

BBQ Sauce	18 oz. Bottle
Butter (bowl/stick)	4 oz./Bowls Vary
Cinnamon	
Cream Cheese	2 oz. Pkgs.
Garlic Powder	2.5 oz. Bottle
Gouda Cheese	4 oz. Tub
Habanera/Hot Sauce	6 oz. Bottle
Hazelnut Spread	7.7 oz. Jar
Jalapeno Peppers	1.3 oz. Singles
Jelly-Grape	12 oz. Bottle
Ketchup	20 oz. Bottle
Mustard	14 oz. Bottle
No-Salt-Seasoning	2.5 oz. Bottle
Onion Powder	2.62 oz Bottle
Peanut Butter	18 oz. Jar
Pickle (Large Dill)	9 oz. Single
Pickle Juice	
Ranch Dressing	2 oz. Pkg.
Salad Dressing	15 oz. Jar
Salsa	8 oz. Bottle
Salt/Pepper	Shakers
Sandwich Spread	15 oz. Jar
Seasoning Packets from Ramen	Single Packets

Squeeze Cheese...16 oz. Bottle
Strawberry Preserves...12 oz. Bottle
Sugar..Cubes
Sweetener...Single Packets

Cookies

Chocolate Chip...12 oz. Package
Chocolate/Duplex/Strawberry/Vanilla Crème.......16 oz. Package
Maria Cookies...5.6 oz. Package
Vanilla Wafers...16 oz. Bag

Drinks

Cappuccino (variety flavors)..........................12 oz. Package
Creamer (variety flavors)...............................12 oz. Bag
Drink Mix (Kool-Aid) (variety flavors) .... .14 oz. (1 Tbsp.)
Electrolytes... .14 oz. Package
Hot Chocolate Mix..10 oz. Bag
Instant Coffee-Columbian..............................4 oz. Bag
Instant Coffee-Plantation...............................4 oz. Bag
Instant Milk..4 oz. Bag
Instant Tea Bags..100 Count Box
Juices/Sodas...12 oz. Cans
Water (cold/hot)
Whey/Chikes(protein powders) (variety flavors)...2 oz. Packages

Meats

Beef Brisket..6 oz. Packages
Chicken Bites...4 oz. Packages
Chicken Chili..8 oz. Packages
Chicken Chunks...7 oz. Packages
Chili with/without Beans.................................11.25 oz. Packages
Mackerel (Regular) ....3.5 oz. Packages
Mackerel (Siracha) ....3.53 oz. Packages
Pink Salmon...5 oz. Packages

Roast Beef..12 oz. Packages
Spam..3 oz. Packages
Summer Sausages...................................5 oz. Packages
Tuna Jalapenos.......................................3.53 oz. Packages
Tuna (Regular) ....4.34 oz. Packages
Turkey Bites...4 oz. Packages

Miscellaneous

Apple..Single
Black Beans..10-16 oz. Bags
Bread
Corn Bread
Energizer/Trail Mix....................................2 oz. Packages
Flour Tortillas..10 oz. Packages
Granola Bars...Singles
Hot/Salted/Unsalted Peanuts....................2 oz. Packages
Instant Chili Beans...................................12 oz. Bag
Instant Oatmeal..10 Packages Box
Instant Potatoes.......................................10 oz. Bag
Instant Rice-Brown..................................6.5 oz. Bag
Instant Rice-White...................................8 oz. Bag
Mega-Omega Trail Mix............................10 oz. Bag
Pasta Shells...9 oz. Bag
Raisins
Raisin Bran Cereal..................................20 oz. Bag
Ramen Noodles (variety of flavors)..........3 oz. Packages
Refried Beans..15 oz. Bag
Sunflower Seeds......................................6 oz. Bag
Veggies from Trays..................................4 oz. Servings

Total Ingredients – 104 Items

Conversion Chart

Liquid Measurements

Gallons	Quarts	Pints	Cups	Fluid Ounces
1 gal.	4 qt.	8 pt.	16 cups	128 fl. oz.
1/2 gal.	2 qt.	4 pt.	8 cups	64 fl. oz.
1/4 gal.	1 qt.	2 pt.	4 cups	32 fl. oz.
1/8 gal.	1/2 qt.	1 pt.	2 cups	16 fl. oz.
1/16 gal.	1/4 qt.	1/2 pt.	1 cup	8 fl. oz.

Dry Measurements

Cups	Tablespoons	Teaspoons	Ounces	Grams
1 cup	16 tbsp.	48 tsp.	8 oz.	229 g.
3/4 cup	12 tbsp.	36 tsp.	6 oz.	171 g.
2/3 cup	10 2/3 tbsp.	32 tsp.	5.34 oz.	152 g.
1/2 cup	8 tbsp.	24 tsp.	4 oz.	114 g.
1/3 cup	5 1/2 tbsp.	16 tsp.	2.67 oz.	76 g.
1/4 cup	4 tbsp.	12 tsp.	2 oz.	57 g.
1/8 cup	2 tbsp.	6 tsp.	1 oz.	29 g.
1/16 cup	1 tbsp.	3 tsp.	.5 oz.	14 g.

1 Coffee Mug = 12 oz.

Other Cookbooks by Troy Traylor:

Cell Block Cookin'
Fine Dining Prison Cookbook
Fine Dining Prison Cookbook 2

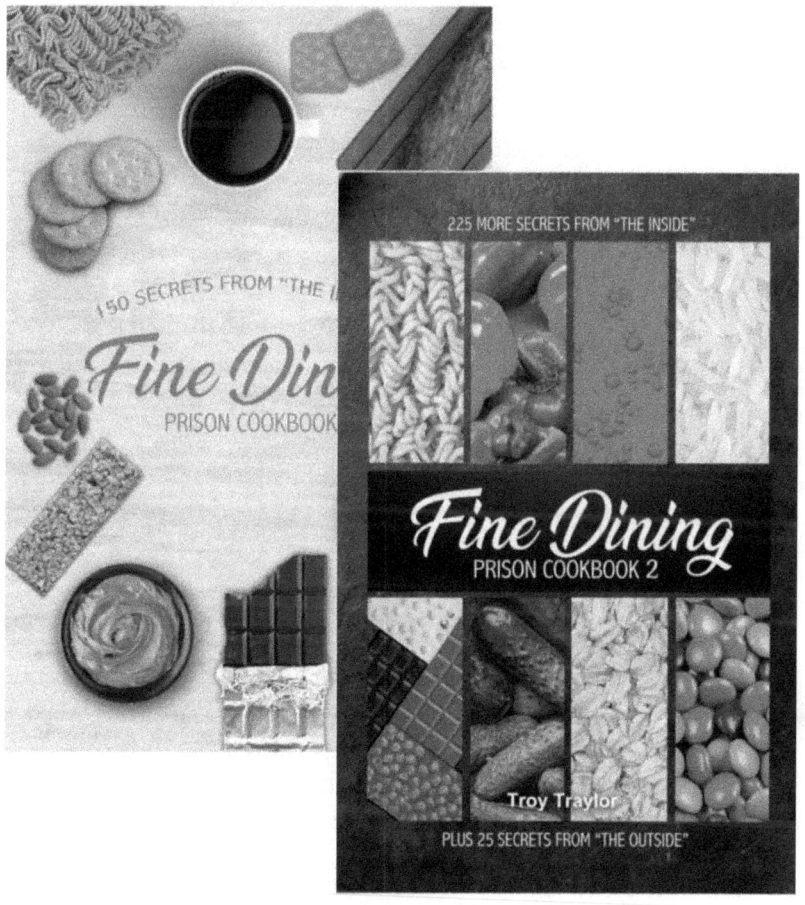

Available Amazon.com and FreebirdPublishers.com

Troy Traylor

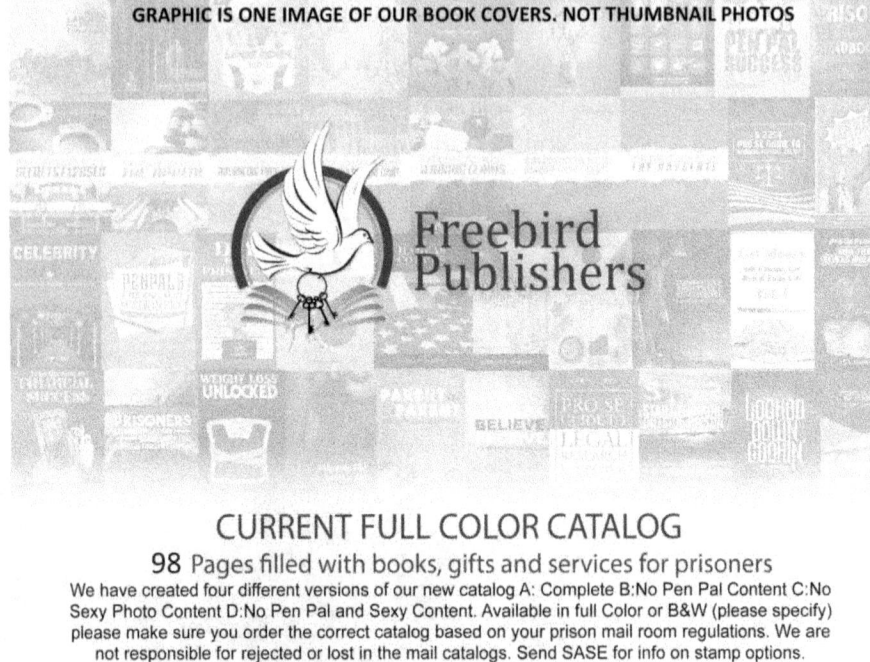

CURRENT FULL COLOR CATALOG
98 Pages filled with books, gifts and services for prisoners

We have created four different versions of our new catalog A: Complete B:No Pen Pal Content C:No Sexy Photo Content D:No Pen Pal and Sexy Content. Available in full Color or B&W (please specify) please make sure you order the correct catalog based on your prison mail room regulations. We are not responsible for rejected or lost in the mail catalogs. Send SASE for info on stamp options.

Freebird Publishers Book Selection Includes:

- Ask. Believe. Receive.: Our Power to Create Our Own Destiny
- Celebrity Female Star Power
- Cell Chef 1 & 2
- Cellpreneur: The Millionaire Prisoner's Guidebook
- Chapter 7 Bankruptcy: Seven Steps to Financial Freedom
- Convicted Creations Cookbook
- Cooking With Hot Water
- DIY for Prisoners
- Federal Rules of Criminal Procedures Pocket Guide
- Federal Rules of Evidence Pocket Guide
- Fine Dining Cookbook 1, 2, 3
- Freebird Publisher's Gift Look Book
- Get Money: Self Educate, Get Rich, & Enjoy Life (3 book series)
- Habeas Corpus Manual
- Hobo Pete and the Ghost Train
- Hot Girl Safari: Non-Nude Photo Book
- How to Write a Good Letter From Prison
- Ineffective Assistance of Counsel
- Inmate Shopper
- Inmate Shopper Censored
- Introduction to Financial Success
- Kitty Kat: Adult Entertainment Resource Book
- Life With a Record
- Locked Down Cookin'
- Locked Up Love Letters: Becoming the Perfect Pen Pal
- Parent to Parent: Raising Children from Prison
- Penacon Presents: The Prisoners Guide to Being a Perfect Pen Pal
- Pen Pal Success: The Ultimate Guide to Getting & Keeping Pen Pals
- Pen Pals: A Personal Guide for Prisoners
- Pillow Talk: Adult Non-Nude Photo Book
- Post-Conviction Relief Series (Books 1-7)
- Prison Health Handbook
- Prison Legal Guide
- Prison Picasso
- Prisoner's Communication Guidelines for Navigating in Prison
- Prisonyland Adult Coloring Book
- Pro Se Guide to Legal Research & Writing
- Pro Se Prisoner: How to Buy Stocks and Bitcoin
- Pro Se Section 1983 Manual
- Section 2254 Pro Se Guide to Winning Federal Relief
- Soft Shots: Adult Non-Nude Photo Book
- The Best 500 Non-Profit Organizations for Prisoners & Their Families
- Weight Loss Unlocked
- Write & Get Paid

PayPal | MasterCard | VISA | DISCOVER | BANK

CATALOG ONLY $5 - SHIPS BY FIRST CLASS MAIL
ADDITIONAL OPTION: add $5 for Shipping and Handling with Tracking

NO ORDER FORM NEEDED CLEARLY WRITE ON PAPER & SEND PAYMENT TO:
FREEBIRD PUBLISHERS 221 Pearl St., Ste. 541, North Dighton, MA 02764
www.FreebirdPublishers.com Diane@FreebirdPublishers.com Text/Phone: 774-406-8682
We accept all forms of payment. Plus Venmo & CashApp! Venmo: @FreebirdPublishers CashApp: $FreebirdPublishers

Fine Dining Prison Cookbook 3

WE NEED YOUR REVIEWS ON amazon

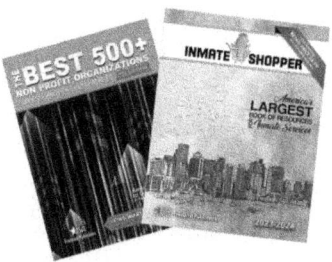

Rate Us & Win!

We do monthly drawings for a FREE copy of one of our publications. Just have your loved one rate any Freebird Publishers book on Amazon and then send us a quick e-mail with your name, inmate number, and institution address and you could win a FREE book.

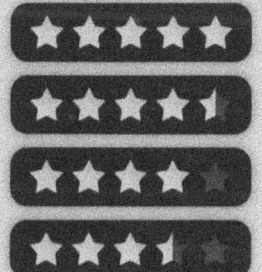

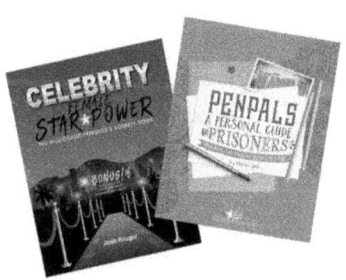

FREEBIRD PUBLISHERS
221 Pearl St., Ste. 541
North Dighton, MA 02764

www.freebirdpublishers.com
Diane@FreebirdPublishers.com

Troy Traylor

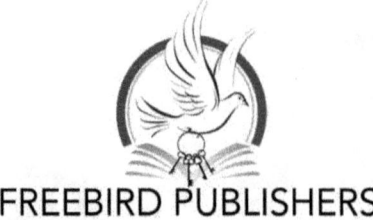

FREEBIRD PUBLISHERS

Thanks for your interest in Freebird Publishers!

We value our customers and would love to hear from you! Reviews are an important part in bringing you quality publications. We love hearing from our readers-rather it's good or bad (though we strive for the best)!

If you could take the time to review/rate any publication you've purchased with Freebird Publishers we would appreciate it!

If your loved one uses Amazon, have them post your review on the books you've read. This will help us tremendously, in providing future publications that are even more useful to our readers and growing our business.

Amazon works off of a 5 star rating system. When having your loved one rate us be sure to give them your chosen star number as well as a written review. Though written reviews aren't required, we truly appreciate hearing from you.

Sample Review Received on Inmate Shopper

 poeticsunshine

★★★★★ **Truly a guide**

Reviewed in the United States on June 29, 2023

Verified Purchase

This book is a powerhouse of information. My son had to calm/ground himself to prioritize where to start.

www.ingramcontent.com/pod-product-compliance
Lightning Source LLC
Chambersburg PA
CBHW070538170426
43200CB00011B/2461